OHNS

OTOLARYNGOLOGY, HEAD AND NECK SURGERY

pocket field guide

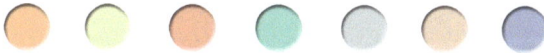

Neil Thomson and Jagdeep Cheema

OHNS pocket field guide

by Neil Thomson and Jagdeep Cheema

© Neil Thomson, 2021. All rights reserved.
ISBN 978-0-6452437-0-3
Published by Neil Thomson.

Book Design and Production by John and Yolande Bull, Publishing Art Australia.
Phone: +61 (02) 4973 1353
Mobile: 0410 622 800 • Email: jnbull2@gmail.com

Printed in Australia by Minuteman Press, Prahran, Victoria.

Creators: Neil Thomson and Jagdeep Cheema, authors.

Title: *OHNS pocket field guide* / Neil Thomson and Jagdeep Cheema.

ISBN 978-0-6452437-0-3 (paperback)

Subjects: Medical / Otolaryngology, Head and Neck Surgery

For further information write: nj.thomson@yahoo.com

A catalogue record for this book is available from the National Library of Australia

DISCLAIMER

The author and publisher have taken all due care in the preparation and publication of this textbook. The reader acknowledges that it has been prepared for educational purposes and is not intended to diagnose, treat, cure or prevent any condition or disease.

This book is not intended as a substitute for consultation with a medical practitioner.

The author and publisher, to the fullest extent, permitted by law, excludes any liability for any consequential loss or damage which may arise in respect of the use of the material in this work.

DEDICATION

To all those in need!

Photo Credits:

Cover and images on pages 10, 22, 50, 60, 70, 82 and 96 by N. Thomson

Photos on pages 4 and 6 by J. Bull

❧

Foreword

This pocket field guide of OHNS is intended to be used either in its paper version or electronically while 'on the run'.

It is aimed at the Medical Student looking for a well-rounded understanding of the conditions of Head and Neck Surgery.

The electronic version is able to give video documentation of the topics under study.

The aim is for students to be able to carry the 'guide' and refer to it in the ED, Ward or Operating Theatre.

Special thanks are extended to John and Yolande Bull for their meticulous work and guidance in preparation of this guidebook.

Thank you also to Richard Davies, audiologist, for his preparation of audiograms and related test results. Gratitude is also extended to our colleagues and friends who have checked, advised and encouraged the compilation of this book.

Thanks to Dr Greg Shein and Elizabeth May for featuring in the Dix-Hallpike Test.

Gratitude is extended to Drs Joyce Ho, Daron Cope, Sebastian Ranguis, James Deeves and Shashinder Singh for their critical analysis and advice.

Dr Neil J. Thomson

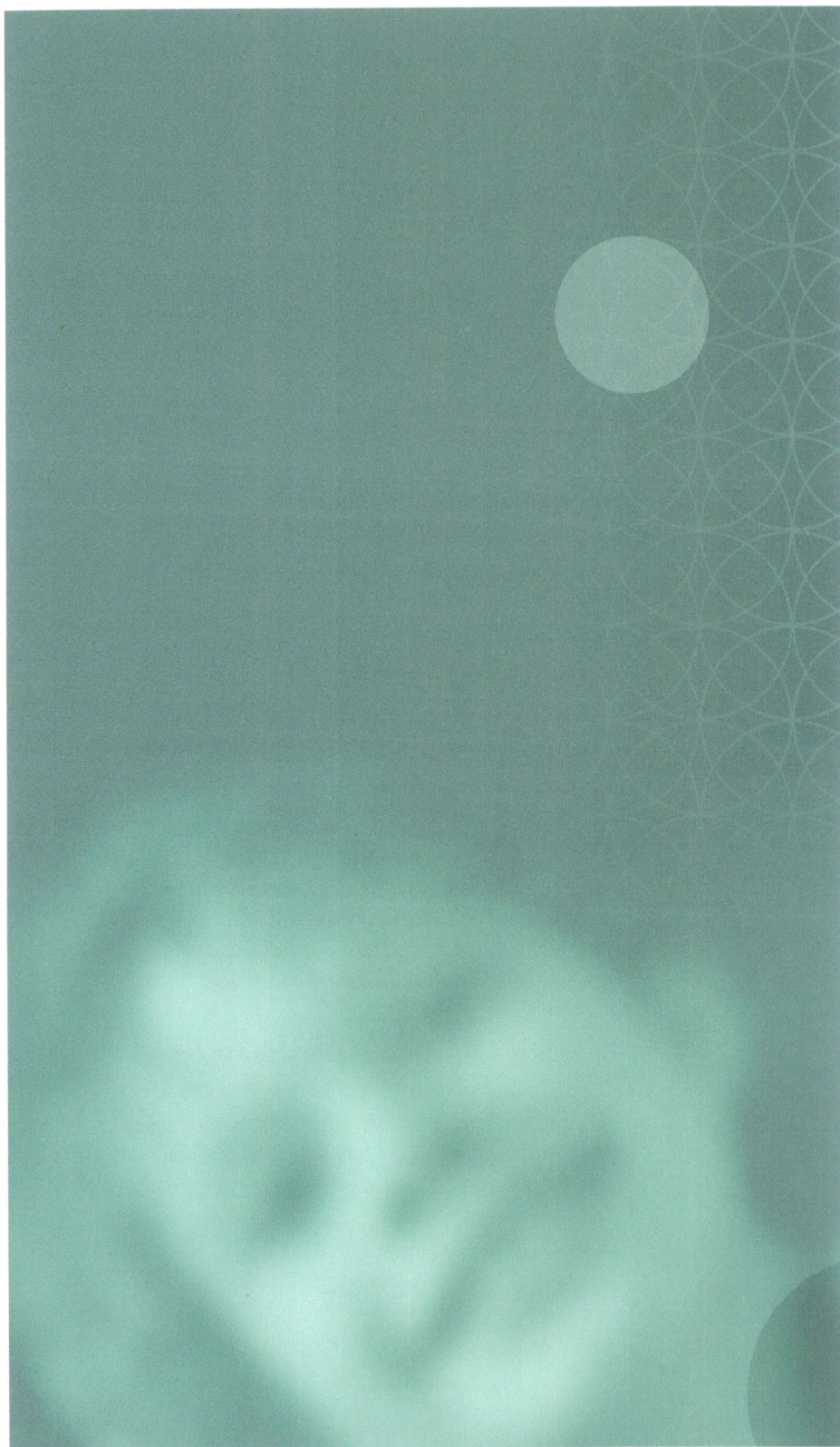

Preface

An introduction to the use of this pocket field guide

This OHNS handbook is designed to give medical students and nurses an overview into the medical and surgical aspects of the speciality.

It is aimed to give as much practical help as possible.

Here there is presentation of what is normal and at the same time, the common pathologies are shown.

There is a strong emphasis on photography as this is a very visual speciality which requires specific equipment to allow a diagnosis to be made.

Contents

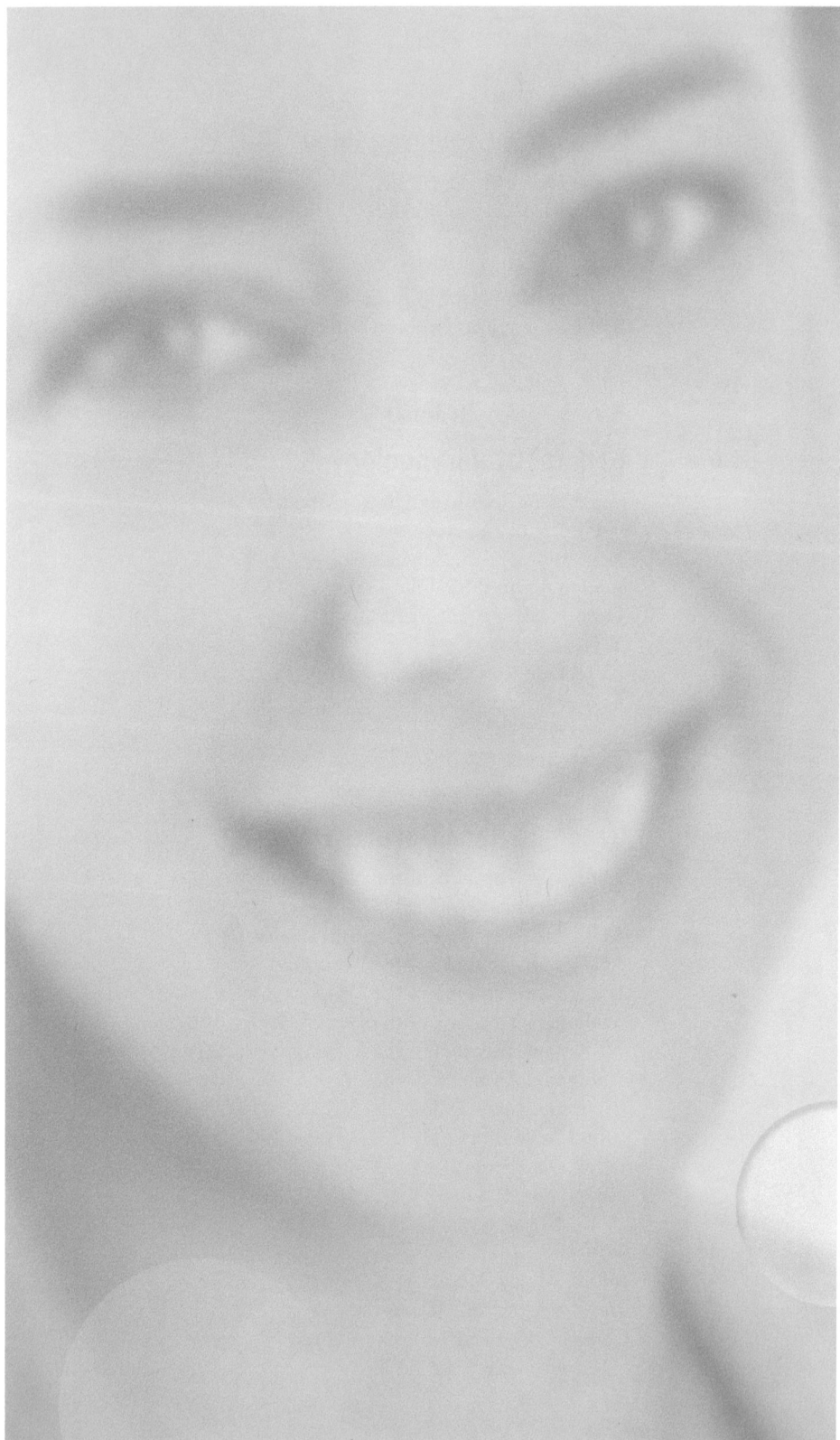

History and Physical Examination

The patient history allows the clinician to gain a general understanding to help formulate a provisional diagnosis. It is vital to put emphasis on the presenting complaints as well as consider the general health of the patient. The physical examination and further investigation will confirm or correct this diagnosis.

HEAD AND NECK SYSTEM REVIEW INCLUDES THE FOLLOWING SYMPTOMS:

Ear	otalgia, otorrhoea, hearing loss, vertigo, tinnitus, fullness
Nose	obstruction, rhinorrhoea, epistaxis, anosmia, facial pressure, post nasal drip
Throat	pain, dysphagia, odynophagia
Larynx	hoarseness, stridor, dyspnoea, odynophonia
Neck	lymphadenopathy, mass, pain
Face	Facial droop

Key Point: Otalgia in the presence of throat/neck symptoms may indicate serious underlying pathology.

INSTRUMENTS

Equipment Necessary:
- Otoscope.
- Tongue depressor.
- Wax hook.
- Jobson-Horne probe.
- Tilley's nasal forceps.
- Crocodile ear forceps.
- Thudicum nasal speculum.
- Tuning fork 512 Hz.
- Light source.
- Ear specula.
- Curettes.
- Nasal and ear suction device.
- Special equipment e.g., flexible nasoendoscope, microscope, tympanometer.

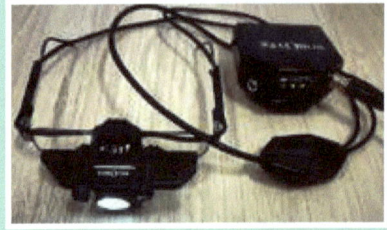

Headlight

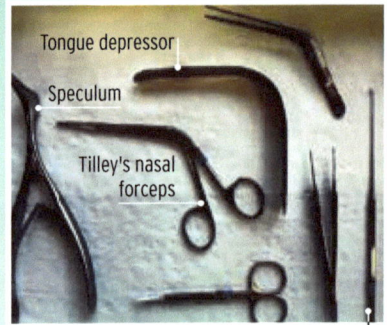

Tongue depressor
Speculum
Tilley's nasal forceps
Jobson-Horne probe

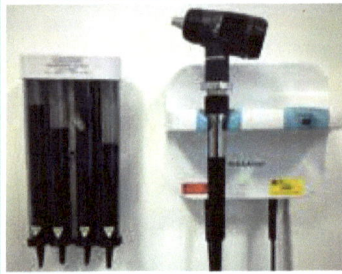

Otoscope

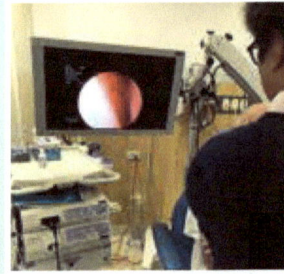

Endoscopic view

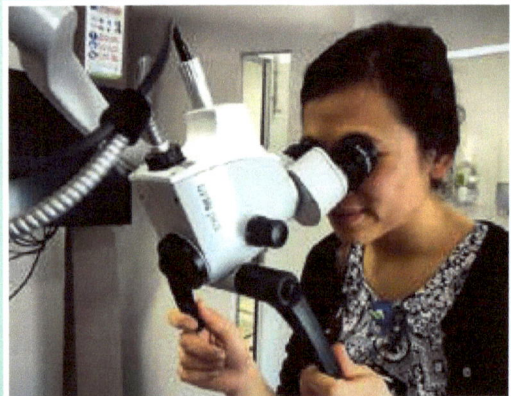

Operating microscope

EXAMINATION OF THE EAR

The External Ear
- Assess the size, shape, position and general condition of the pinnae.
- Examine the post-auricular and mastoid regions for any surgical scars, swelling, erythema, tenderness, masses or congenital anomalies (e.g., pre-auricular pits and sinuses, skin tags).

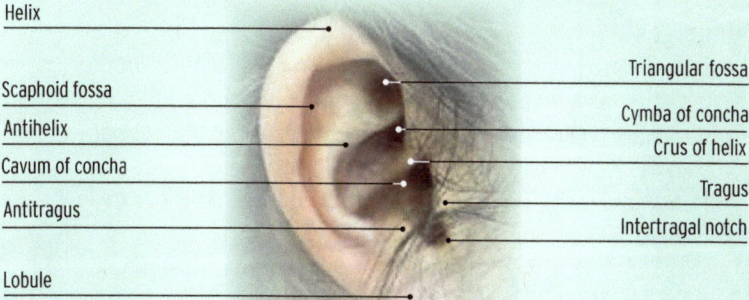

Helix

Scaphoid fossa

Antihelix

Cavum of concha

Antitragus

Lobule

Triangular fossa

Cymba of concha

Crus of helix

Tragus

Intertragal notch

Otoscopy
- Used to assess the ear canal and tympanic membrane. It may be necessary to remove any occluding cerumen.
- Inspect the ear canal for patency, cleanliness, presence of draining lesions or foreign material.
- Assess the tympanic membrane for:
    - Landmarks (handle and lateral process of malleus, incus, pars tensa, pars flaccida, light reflex).
    - Colour.
    - Transparency.
    - Any abnormal findings (bulging, retraction, perforation).
- The mobility of the eardrum can be assessed with pneumatic otoscopy.

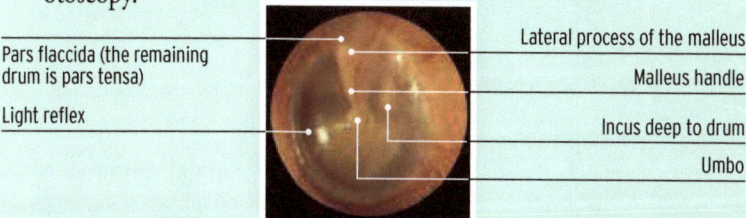

Pars flaccida (the remaining drum is pars tensa)

Light reflex

Lateral process of the malleus

Malleus handle

Incus deep to drum

Umbo

Tuning Fork Tests
- Tuning fork testing is a quick, simple bedside tool that is useful to assess hearing loss.
- Two most common tuning fork tests performed are the Weber Test and the Rinne Test. A 512 Hz tuning fork is used for both.

Weber Test

- Is performed by striking the tuning fork and placing it in the centre of the patient's forehead with firm pressure.
- With normal hearing, the sound radiates to both ears equally.
- With conductive hearing loss, the sound appears louder in the impaired ear.
- With sensorineural hearing loss, the sound appears quieter in the impaired ear.

Rinne Test

- Is performed by striking the tuning fork and placing it on the patient's mastoid process to assess bone conduction. Once it can no longer be heard, the tuning fork is held at the entrance of the ear canal to assess air conduction.
- If AC>BC – this is a positive Rinne Test result. This occurs in normal ears or sensorineural hearing loss.
- If BC>AC – this is a negative Rinne Test result. This occurs in conductive hearing loss.

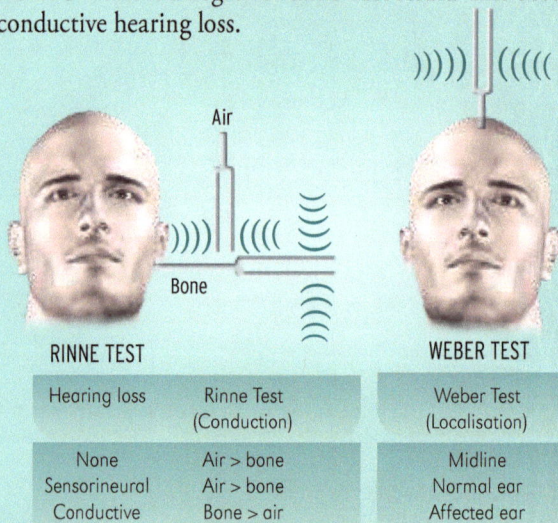

RINNE TEST   WEBER TEST

Hearing loss	Rinne Test (Conduction)	Weber Test (Localisation)
None	Air > bone	Midline
Sensorineural	Air > bone	Normal ear
Conductive	Bone > air	Affected ear

Both tests need to be done in conjunction to give the best interpretation

Otoscopy Examination Tips

- Choose the largest speculum that will fit comfortably in the patient's ear canal.
- Gently pull the pinna upwards and backwards to straighten the ear canal (backwards in children).
- Grip the otoscope like a pen (resting your little finger on the patient's zygomatic arch), using your left hand to examine the left ear and your right hand to examine the right ear.

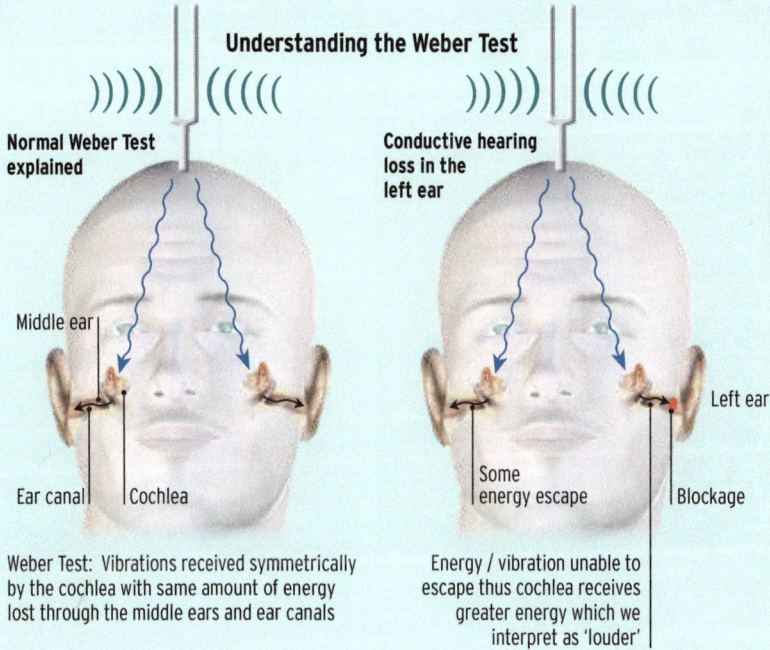

Understanding the Weber Test

Normal Weber Test explained

Conductive hearing loss in the left ear

Middle ear

Left ear

Ear canal | Cochlea

Some energy escape | Blockage

Weber Test: Vibrations received symmetrically by the cochlea with same amount of energy lost through the middle ears and ear canals

Energy / vibration unable to escape thus cochlea receives greater energy which we interpret as 'louder'

EXAMINATION OF THE NOSE

- Inspect the shape of the nose (septal deviation, symmetry of nares), the condition of overlying skin, deformities, presence of any masses or evidence of trauma.
- Assess airway patency by occluding each nostril in turn and observe breathing through the opposite side. Breathing should be silent at rest. Also look for alar collapse (collapse of the nasal soft tissues during inspiration). This can also be tested by holding a cold shiny surface (e.g., metal tongue depressor) under the nose and looking for condensation on the metal surface during expiration.
- Elevate the nasal tip and examine the nasal vestibule. Next, insert a nasal speculum to evaluate the mucosa, nasal septum, floor of the nose and the turbinates (inferior and middle).
- Examination of the posterior nasal cavity and postnasal space requires a nasoendoscope.

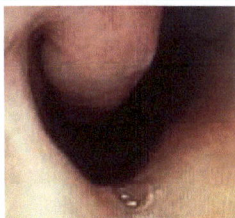

Right nostril with the inferior turbinate, centrally attached to the lateral wall with the septum on the opposite side

EXAMINATION OF THE ORAL CAVITY

Examination of the oral cavity and oropharynx should include an assessment of the following structures:

Lips
- Assess colour, symmetry and examine for any lesions.

Gingiva, Teeth and Buccal Mucosa
- Using a tongue depressor to lift each cheek away from the teeth, assess the condition of the gingivae, teeth, buccal mucosa and the parotid duct orifices (opposite the upper second molar). Also examine beneath the upper and lower lips.

Tongue and Floor of the Mouth
- Examine the mucosa and mobility of the tongue and note any masses or ulcers. Ensure to inspect all surfaces of the tongue as well as the floor of the mouth for the orifices of the submandibular ducts (just lateral to the frenulum).

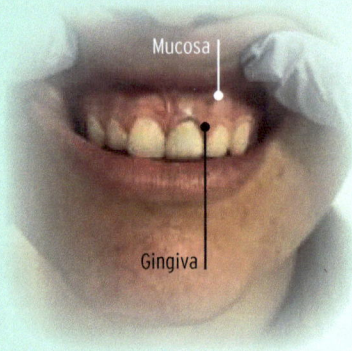

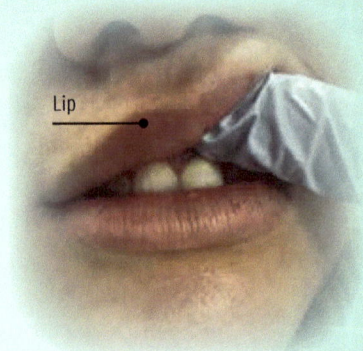

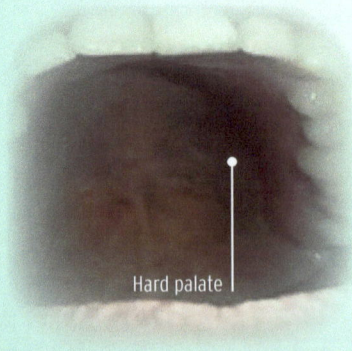

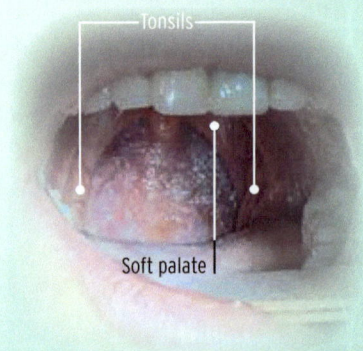

- It is important to palpate the tongue, including the tongue base, as small surface lesions may have extensive submucosal extension.

Submandibular Glands

- Palpate the glands bimanually. Place one finger on the floor of the mouth and the other hand below the angle of the mandible.
- The glands should be mobile, non-tender and of equal size.

Oropharynx and Palate

- Depress the anterior half of the tongue to examine the palatine tonsils and the anterior and posterior pillars.
- Inspect the hard and soft palates for any lesions. Assess the symmetry and movements of the soft palate.

Ensure to examine 'coffins corner' (medial to the molars).

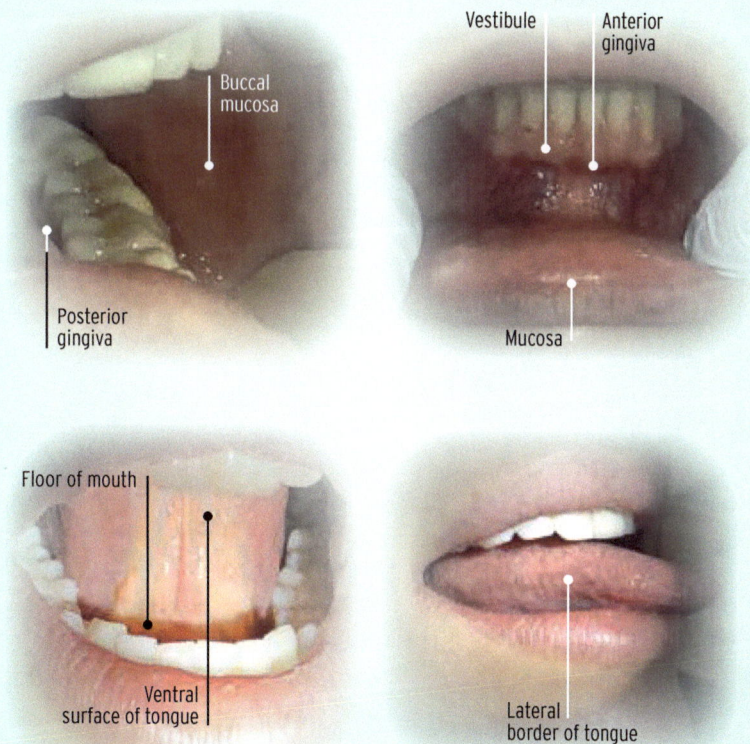

Buccal mucosa

Posterior gingiva

Vestibule

Anterior gingiva

Mucosa

Floor of mouth

Ventral surface of tongue

Lateral border of tongue

EXAMINATION OF THE LARYNX

Examination is important to perform in any patient with a voice disorder, throat pain, painful swallowing, neck mass or referred otalgia. Inspection is performed with a flexible laryngoscope.

Flexible Endoscopy
- Spray a small amount of topical anaesthesia into the nostril.
- Insert the scope into the nostril and examine the structures on the way to the larynx.
- Assess the nasal cavity mucosa, turbinates, Eustachian tube orifice and look for nasal or nasopharyngeal masses. Examine the oropharynx and hypopharynx for any abnormalities.
- Larynx: Inspect the supraglottic structures (epiglottis, aryepiglottic folds, arytenoid cartilages and false vocal folds) and glottis (true vocal folds). Inspect the appearance of the mucosa and assess for symmetry and vocal fold mobility on inspiration and phonation.

Relation of Hyoid Bone, Thyroid Cartilage, Trachea and Thyroid Gland
(Note: Small abnormal nodule on the right lobe)

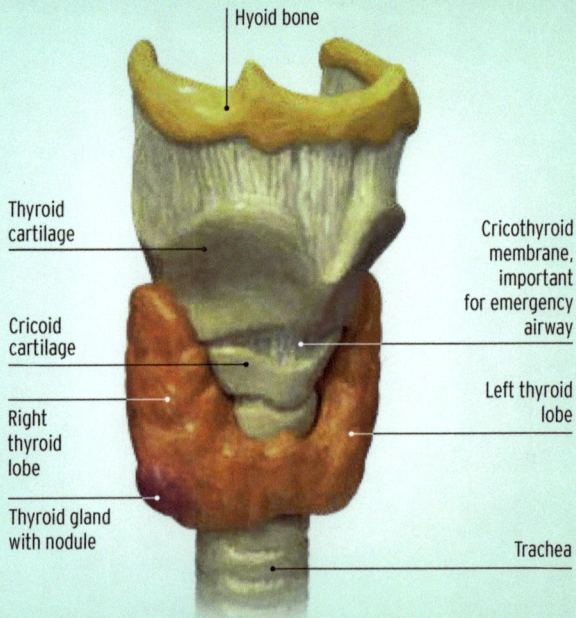

Hyoid bone

Thyroid cartilage

Cricothyroid membrane, important for emergency airway

Cricoid cartilage

Left thyroid lobe

Right thyroid lobe

Thyroid gland with nodule

Trachea

EXAMINATION OF THE NECK

- Inspect from the front of the patient for any visible masses, scars, skin discolouration or other abnormalities.
- Palpate the neck from behind the patient and should include examination of the anterior and posterior triangles, larynx, thyroid gland, supraclavicular area and lymph nodes.
- If the patient has an obvious mass, begin the examination there:
  - Comment on location, size, colour, mobility, tenderness, consistency, pulsatility and fixation to adjacent structures.
  - Ask patient to swallow and stick out their tongue.
  - Watch for movement of any masses.
- A systematic sequence for examining the rest of the neck is important to avoid missing another mass.

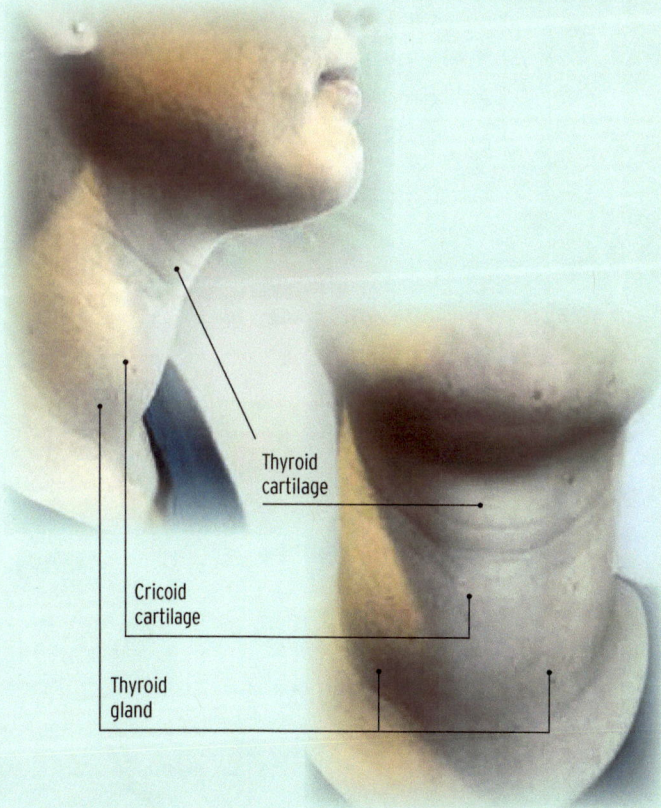

Thyroid cartilage

Cricoid cartilage

Thyroid gland

Normal neck structures - slight symmetric fullness of the thyroid often seen in younger females.

EXAMINATION OF CRANIAL NERVES

It is important to assess the function of the cranial nerves in a head and neck examination.

CRANIAL NERVE	TESTING
CN I	Smell sensation of each nostril separately
CN II	Visual acuity of each eye separately
CN III, IV, VI	Extraocular motility
CN V	Sensation over the 3 divisions (forehead, cheek, mentum); muscles of mastication
CN VII	See below – facial nerve function
CN VIII	Tuning forks/whisper testing
CN IX, X	Sensation of posterior third of tongue; assessing palatal elevation, vocal cord function and swallowing
CN XI	Sternocleidomastoid and trapezius muscle strength
CN XII	Integrity of motor nerve supply to tongue

Facial Nerve Function
- Examine general appearance of patient.
- Ask patient to:
  - Raise their eyebrows.
  - Shut their eyes tightly.
  - Flare their nostrils.
  - Blow out their cheeks.
  - Smile and form a whistle.
- Grade the patient's facial weakness using the 'House-Brackmann Facial Nerve Grading System'.

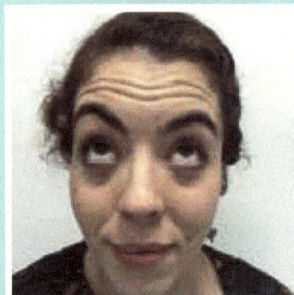

Crease up the forehead

FACIAL WEAKNESS GRADING – (HOUSE–BRACKMANN)

GRADE	DESCRIPTION	GROSS FUNCTION	RESTING APPEARANCE	DYNAMIC APPEARANCE
1	Normal	Normal	Normal	Normal
2	Mild dysfunction	Slight weakness with effort, may have mild synkinesis	Normal	Mild oral and forehead asymmetry, complete eye closure with minimal effort
3	Moderate dysfunction	Obvious asymmetry with movement, noticeable synkinesis	Normal	Mild oral asymmetry, complete eye closure with effort, slight forehead movement
4	Moderately severe dysfunction	Obvious asymmetry, disfiguring asymmetry	Normal	Asymmetrical mouth, incomplete eye closure, no forehead movement
5	Severe dysfunction	Barely perceptible movement	Asymmetric	Slight oral/nasal movement with effort, incomplete eye closure
6	Total paralysis	None	Asymmetric	No movement

Reference: House J.W. Brackmann D.E. Facial Nerve Grading System. Otolaryngol Head Neck Surg 1985; 93: 146 –147.

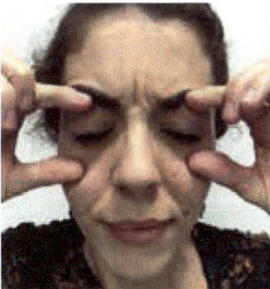

Keep eyes closed against resistance

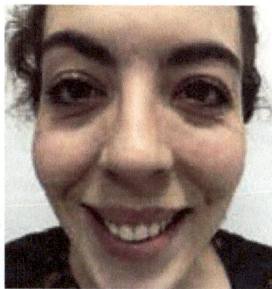

Reveal the teeth

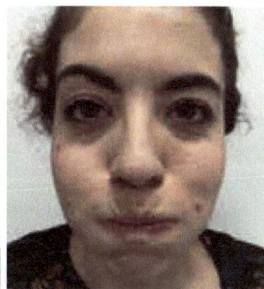

Puff out the cheeks

CHAPTER 2

Otology

*The study of the ear in all of its three parts
– external, middle and inner ear.*

*This is the structure of hearing and contains
a crucial balance control mechanism.*

ANATOMY OF THE EAR

The ear is divided into three parts: The external, middle and inner ear.

The External Ear is made up of:

Pinna
- Consists of elastic cartilage surrounded by skin on either side. Acts to funnel sound waves into the external auditory canal.

External Auditory Canal (EAC)
- Consists of a lateral cartilaginous portion and a medial bony portion. Transmits sound waves to the tympanic membrane.

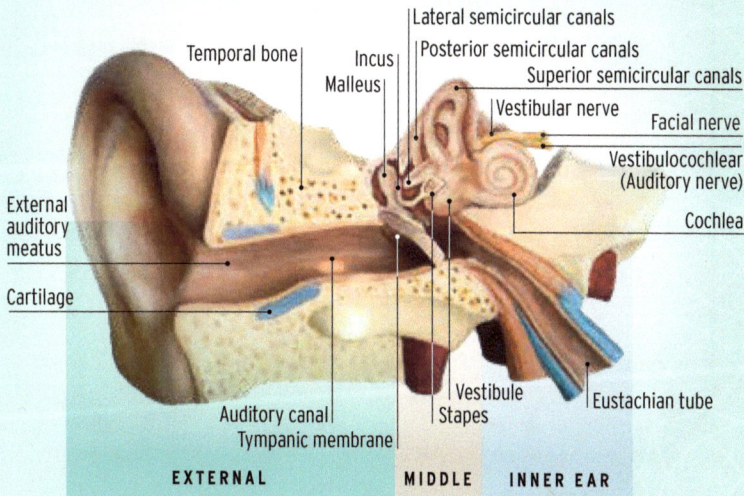

Labels on figure:
Temporal bone · Incus · Malleus · Lateral semicircular canals · Posterior semicircular canals · Superior semicircular canals · Vestibular nerve · Facial nerve · Vestibulocochlear (Auditory nerve) · Cochlea · External auditory meatus · Cartilage · Auditory canal · Tympanic membrane · Vestibule · Stapes · Eustachian tube · EXTERNAL · MIDDLE · INNER EAR

See also Cross-section of the Cochlea, Endnotes Page 115

The Middle Ear is made up of:

Tympanic Membrane (TM)
- Oval shaped and composed of three layers – outer squamous, middle fibrous layer and inner mucosa.

Middle Ear Cavity
- Medial to the tympanic membrane, it is an air containing space that houses the ossicles – malleus, incus and stapes. It is connected to the nasopharynx via the Eustachian tube and to the mastoid air cells via the aditus.

The Inner Ear:
- The inner ear is made up of the cochlea and the vestibular system with the semicircular canals.

PHYSIOLOGY OF HEARING

Events Involved in Hearing

1 Sound waves arrive at the tympanic membrane.

2 Movement of the tympanic membrane causes the displacement of auditory ossicles.

3 Movement of the stapes at the oval window establishes pressure waves in the perilymph of the vestibular duct.

4 The pressure waves distort the basilar membrane on their way to the round window of the tympanic duct.

5 Vibration of the basilar membrane causes vibration of the hair cells against the tectorial membrane.

6 Information about the region and the intensity of the situation is relayed to the CNS over the cochlea branch of the cranial nerve VIII.

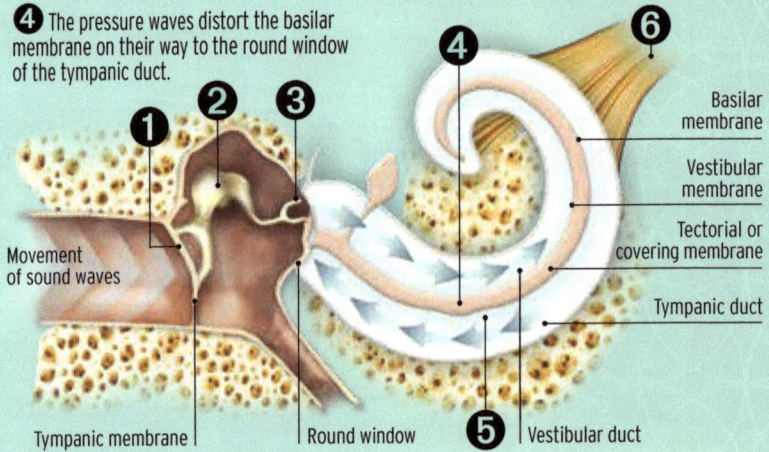

Basilar membrane

Vestibular membrane

Tectorial or covering membrane

Tympanic duct

Movement of sound waves

Tympanic membrane | Round window **5** | Vestibular duct

Ascending Pathway of Hearing
Key Points:

- Information from each ear passes to both sides of the brain which gives some protection in brain injuries.

- The auditory cortex is arranged according to the frequency of energy to the ear.

The adjacent diagram is a simplified summary of the hearing pathway which consists of four relays with fast myelinated fibres. It is interesting to note that each relay nucleus has a specific function of decoding and integration e.g.:

1. Cochlea nucleus – intensity and frequency.

2. Superior olivary complex with sound localisation.

3. Inferior colliculus – localisation of sound.

4. Medial geniculate ganglion – prepare for a verbal response.

Note: Auditory cortex – message recognition and memorising.

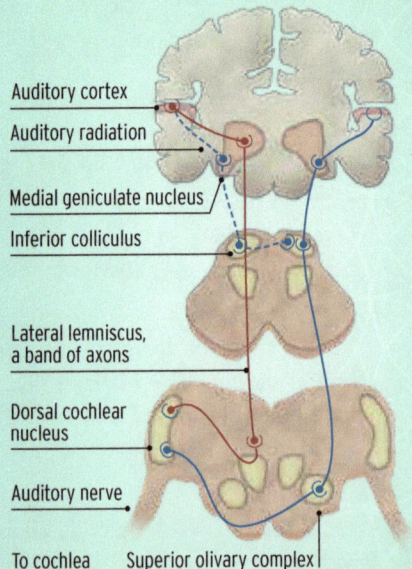

Auditory cortex

Auditory radiation

Medial geniculate nucleus

Inferior colliculus

Lateral lemniscus, a band of axons

Dorsal cochlear nucleus

Auditory nerve

To cochlea   Superior olivary complex

TYPES OF HEARING LOSS

1. Conductive Hearing Loss
- Interference of the conduction of sound to the cochlea.
- Can be caused by external and middle ear diseases.

2. Sensorineural Hearing Loss (SNHL)
- Defect in the conversion of sound energy into nerve impulses or in the transmission of those nerve impulses to the cortex.

3. Mixed Hearing Loss
- Both a conductive hearing loss and a sensorineural hearing loss are present.

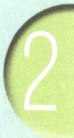

AUDIOLOGIC TESTING

PURE TONE AUDIOMETRY
Provides measurements of hearing level thresholds by air conduction (AC) and bone conduction (BC). A threshold is the softest intensity level at which a patient can hear the tone 50% of the time. Thresholds are obtained for each ear for frequencies from 250 to 8000 Hz.

Air conduction thresholds are obtained with headphones and measure the outer ear, middle ear, inner ear and auditory nerve function.

Bone conduction thresholds are obtained with bone conduction oscillators, which bypass the outer and middle ear.

PURE TONE PATTERNS

1. Conductive Hearing Loss
- BC in normal range.
- AC outside of normal range.
- Gap between AC and BC thresholds is >10 dB (an air-bone gap).

2. Sensorineural Hearing Loss
- Both AC and BC thresholds below normal.
- Gap between AC and BC thresholds is <10 dB (no air-bone gap).

3. Mixed Hearing Loss
- Both AC and BC thresholds below normal.
- Gap between AC and BC thresholds is >10 dB (an air-bone gap).

Conductive Hearing Loss
Hearing is better through bone than through air

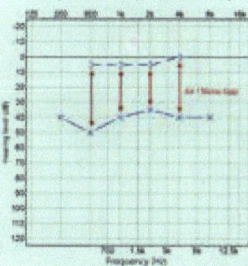

Bilateral Sensorineural Hearing Loss in the higher frequencies

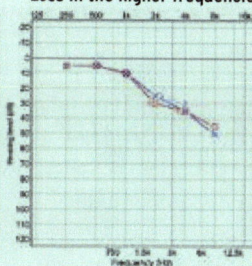

Mixed Hearing Loss

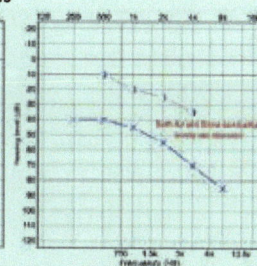

TYMPANOMETRY

- Measures the compliance of the middle ear system.
- A pure tone signal is fed into a sealed external auditory canal and the reflected sound levels are measured at different pressures ranging from –400 to +200 mm of water.
- Tympanogram peak occurs at the point of maximum compliance, where the pressure in the external ear canal is equivalent to the pressure in the middle ear.
- Normal range is between –100 and +50 mm of water.

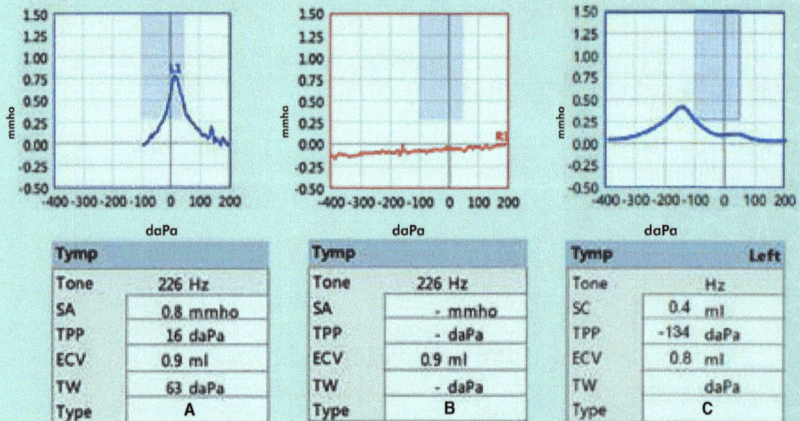

Tymp	
Tone	226 Hz
SA	0.8 mmho
TPP	16 daPa
ECV	0.9 ml
TW	63 daPa
Type	A

Tymp	
Tone	226 Hz
SA	- mmho
TPP	- daPa
ECV	0.9 ml
TW	- daPa
Type	B

Tymp	Left
Tone	Hz
SC	0.4 ml
TPP	-134 daPa
ECV	0.8 ml
TW	daPa
Type	C

Type A	Normal tympanogram (also seen in SNHL)
Type B	Restricted TM mobility (e.g., fluid in the middle ear or TM perforation)
Type C	Significant negative pressure in the ear (e.g., Eustachian tube dysfunction, May have fluid/air bubbles in the middle ear)

OTOACOUSTIC EMISSIONS

- Objective test of hearing where a series of clicks is presented to the ear and the cochlea generates an echo which can be measured.
- Often used in newborn screening.
- Absence of emissions can be due to hearing loss from the inner ear or fluid in the middle ear.

ABR testing (Auditory Brainstem Response)

This test is carried out in those who cannot complete a typical hearing test. Electrodes are placed on the skin over the head and brainwaves are recorded as a response to sounds from headphones. The test can also be used as a screening test for newborn babies. The screening test is set at one level of loudness and the result is either a pass or fail. If test has failed then other testing will be undertaken.

DISEASES OF THE EXTERNAL EAR

OTITIS EXTERNA (OE)

Definition
- Inflammation of the external auditory canal.

Epidemiology
- Occurs in all age groups. • Higher prevalence in the warmer months.

Aetiology

Causative Agents
- Bacteria – Pseudomonas aeruginosa, Staphylococcus epidermidis, Staphylococcus aureus.
- Fungal – Candida albicans.

Risk Factors
- Water exposure.
- Devices occluding the EAC (e.g., earphones, hearing aids).
- Trauma to skin lining the external auditory canal.

Clinical Presentation
- Otalgia, otorrhoea, hearing loss.
- Tenderness with auricle traction or tragal pressure.
- Erythematous and oedematous external auditory canal.
- If severe, fever and post-auricular lymphadenopathy present.

Diagnosis
- Clinical diagnosis guided by history and physical examination.

Treatment
- Clean the external auditory canal of cerumen and purulent material. This is done under a microscope aided by suction.
- Treatment of the infection with topical agents – antibiotics, antiseptics, antifungals and/or steroids.
  - Eardrops are generally used in mild disease, however, if severe canal occlusion, a wick can be inserted.
  - Oral/intravenous antibiotics can be combined if the patient is immunocompromised or evidence of deep tissue infection.
- Analgesia if otalgia present.

Complications
- Periauricular cellulitis.
- Malignant otitis externa.

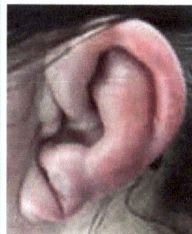

Infective cellulitis from otitis externa

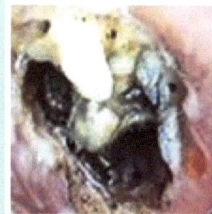

Fungal otitis externa

MALIGNANT (NECROTISING) OTITIS EXTERNA

Definition
- Osteomyelitis of the temporal bone.

Epidemiology
- Population at risk include the elderly, diabetics and immuno-compromised patients.

Aetiology
- Rare complication of otitis externa.
- Causative agent: Pseudomonas aeruginosa in 95% of patients.

Clinical Presentation
- Otalgia and otorrhea that is unresponsive to topical agents used in otitis externa.
- Granulation tissue may be present on the floor of the EAC.

Investigation
- Swab otorrhea for gram stain and culture.
- Imaging: CT scan and MRI of temporal bone; Gallium scan and bone scan.

Treatment
- IV antibiotics – antipseudomonal.
- Hyperbaric oxygen (for consideration).
- May require debridement.

Complications
- Cranial nerve involvement (most commonly facial nerve).
- Meningitis.
- Brain abscess.
- Dural sinus thrombophlebitis.

Key Point: Called malignant because of its aggressiveness and the seriousness of the infection. It is not a cancer.

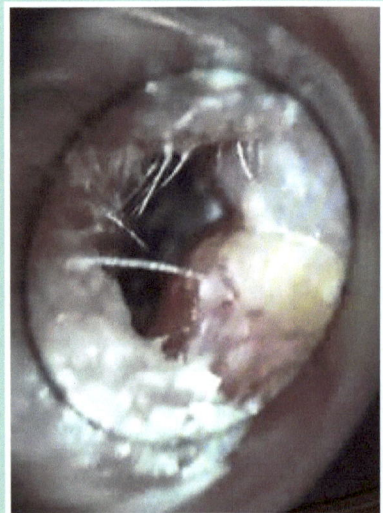

Malignant otitis externa with canal granulation tissue

CERUMEN IMPACTION

Definition
- Cerumen (also known as ear wax) is a naturally produced protective covering in the ear canal. Cerumen is a combination of sebaceous secretions, ceruminous secretions, desquamated skin and immunoglobulins.
- Excessive cerumen accumulation in the ear canal can lead to impaction.

Aetiology
- Cerumen overproduction.
- Narrowing of the ear canal.
- Ear canal disease leading to obstruction.

Risk Factors
- Cotton buds.
- Hearing aids.
- Ear plugs.

Clinical Presentation
- May be asymptomatic if mild.
- Hearing loss, otalgia, ear fullness, vertigo, tinnitus.

Diagnosis
- History and direct visualisation on otoscopic examination.

Treatment
- Cerumenolytics (wax softening agents).
- Irrigation.
- Manual debridement.

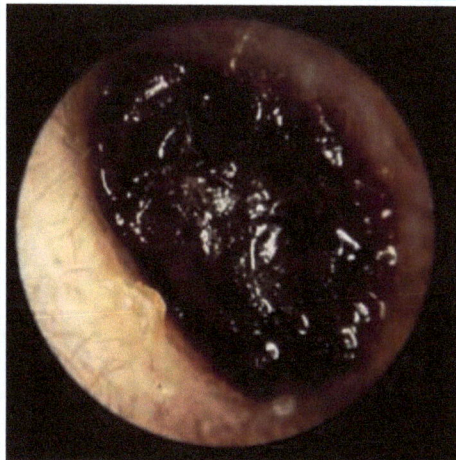

Wax occlusion of ear canal

EXOSTOSES

Definition
- Benign bony outgrowth of the ear canal.

Epidemiology
- Increased prevalence in the surfer population.

Aetiology
- Irritation to the ear canal from repeated exposure to cold water or wind.

Clinical Presentation
- Usually asymptomatic unless large.
- Hearing loss, otitis externa, cerumen impaction.

Investigation
- Audiogram.
- CT scan.

Treatment
- Surgical removal of exostoses if large and symptomatic.

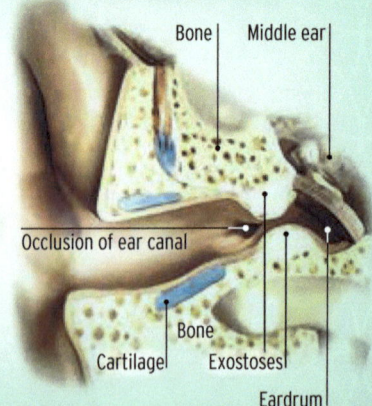

Exostoses partially occluding the ear canal

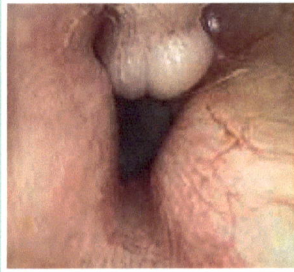

Cross-section of the Normal Ear

Bone | Middle ear

External auditory canal (ear canal)

Bone

Cartilage

Eardrum (tympanic membrane)

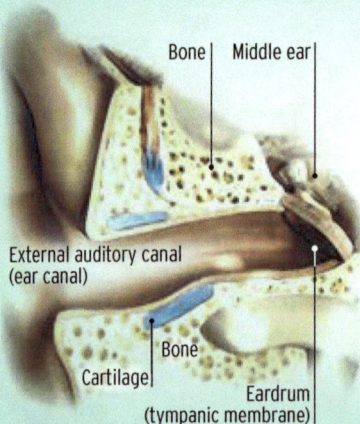

Cross-section of Exostoses and Occluded Ear Canal

Bone | Middle ear

Occlusion of ear canal

Bone

Cartilage | Exostoses

Eardrum

DISEASES OF THE MIDDLE EAR

1. ACUTE OTITIS MEDIA (AOM) AND OTITIS MEDIA WITH EFFUSION (OME)
See also Paediatric Otolaryngology Chapter 5, Page 70

2. CHOLESTEATOMA

Definition
- Abnormal growth of keratinising squamous epithelium in the middle ear and mastoid. It may progressively enlarge destroying adjacent structures (e.g., ossicles).

Classification
- Congenital:
  - Develops as a small white mass behind an intact tympanic membrane in a child with no history of middle ear disease.
- Acquired (more common):
  - Develops after birth as a consequence of chronic middle ear disease.

Pathophysiology
- Acquired:
  - Usually arises due to retraction pockets forming in the pars flaccida, trapping desquamating cells leading to the formation of a cholesteatoma.
  - Less commonly, they form through marginal perforations of the tympanic membrane or through temporal bone fractures.

Risk factors
- History of recurrent AOM and OME.
- Craniofacial anomalies.
- Down Syndrome.
- Cleft palate.

Clinical Presentation
- Progressive hearing loss.
- Otalgia, otorrhea, ear fullness, fever.
- Otoscopy may reveal: Retraction pocket in TM, TM perforation, granulation tissue.

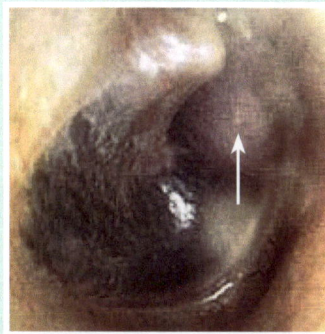

Pale white /pink congenital cholesteotoma in a 2 year old

Investigation
- Audiogram.
- CT scan.

Treatment
- Surgical: Tympanomastoidectomy.

COMPLICATIONS – DISEASES OF THE MIDDLE EAR

EXTRACRANIAL	INTRACRANIAL
Conductive hearing loss (ossicular erosion) or sensorineural hearing loss (inner ear erosion)	Meningitis
Mastoiditis	Brain abscess
Facial nerve palsy	Sigmoid sinus thrombosis

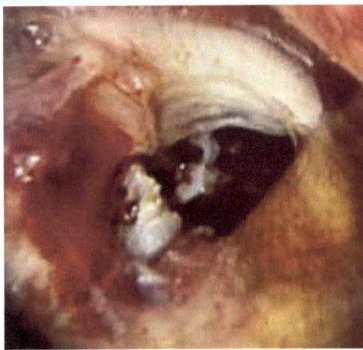

Cholesteatoma
in the middle ear
with perforation

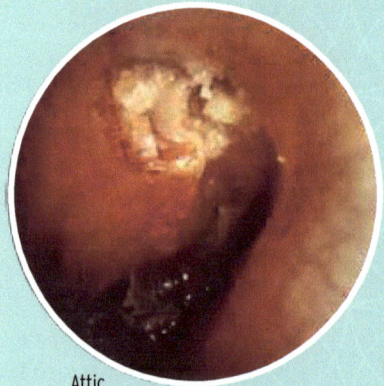

Attic
cholesteatoma

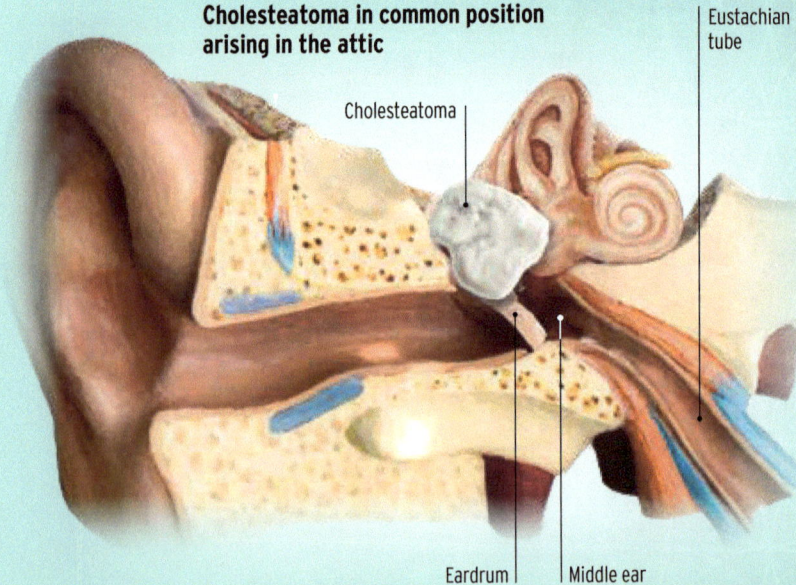

Cholesteatoma in common position arising in the attic

Eustachian tube

Cholesteatoma

Eardrum

Middle ear

MASTOIDITIS

Definition
- Inflammation of the mastoid air cells.
- Epidemiology.
- Occurs more commonly in children than adults.

Aetiology
- Complication of AOM.
- Causative agents: Same as AOM (Streptococcus pneumoniae, H. influenzae, M. catarrhalis).

Pathophysiology
- The middle ear cavity is continuous with the mastoid air cells. During an episode of AOM, the inflammation can spread into the mucosal lining of the mastoid air cells causing mastoiditis.

Clinical Presentation
- Otalgia, otorrhea, hearing loss.
- Lethargy, fever.
- Postauricular tenderness, erythema and swelling.
- Protrusion of the ear.

Investigation
- Imaging: CT scan temporal bone (showing opacification of mastoid air cells).

Treatment
- IV antibiotics.
- Myringotomy and ventilation tube.
- Indications for surgery (mastoidectomy):
    - Failure of medical treatment.
    - Symptoms of intracranial complications.

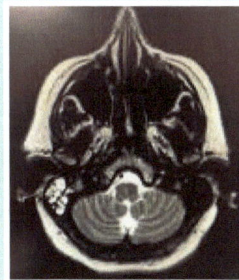

Right ear mastoiditis on MR scan

COMPLICATIONS

EXTRACRANIAL	INTRACRANIAL
Subperiosteal abscess	Meningitis
Facial nerve palsy	Brain abscess
Osteomyelitis	Venous sinus thrombosis
Bezold abscess	
Labyrinthitis	

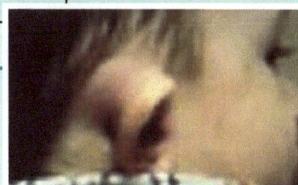

Mastoiditis in a child
(ear pushed anteriorly with
high postauricular swelling)

OTOSCLEROSIS

Definition

- Bony overgrowth of the stapes footplate leading to stapes fixation and conductive hearing loss.

Epidemiology

- More common in women.
- Occurs more frequently between the ages of 20 to 50.

Aetiology

- Cause unknown but represents a disorder of bone growth.
- Possible genetic predisposition.

Clinical Presentation

- Slow, progressive hearing loss (in one or both ears).
- Tinnitus may be present.
- Otoscopy: Normal TM; Increased vascularity of the middle ear bony prominence may be seen through the TM (Schwartz's Sign).

Investigation

- Audiogram: Shows conductive hearing loss. Depression in the bone conduction audiogram at 2 kHz (Carhart's Notch) is a characteristic feature.

Treatment

- Hearing aids.
- Stapedectomy or stapedotomy with a prosthesis is definitive treatment.

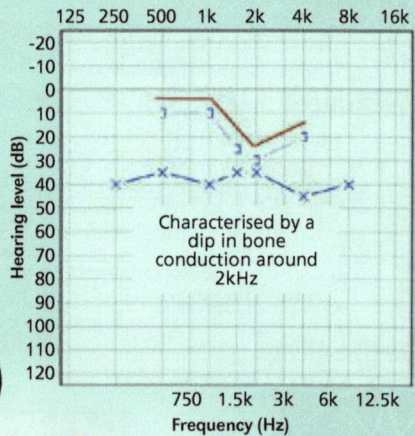

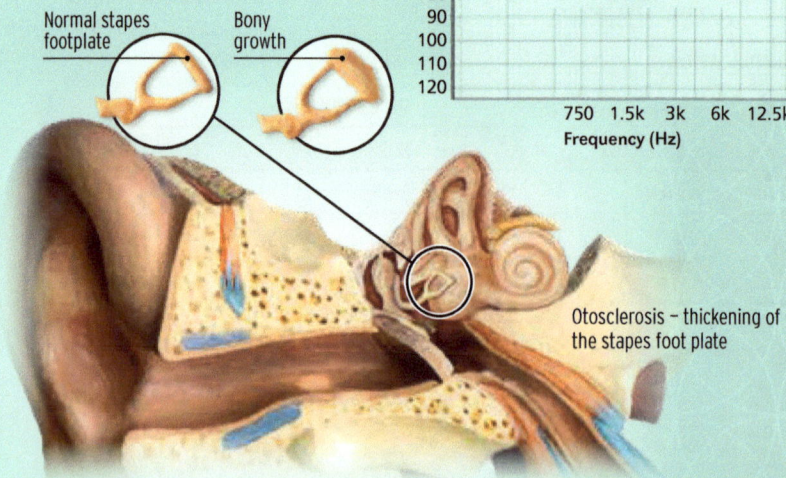

Characterised by a dip in bone conduction around 2kHz

Normal stapes footplate

Bony growth

Otosclerosis – thickening of the stapes foot plate

DISEASES OF THE INNER EAR

CONGENITAL SENSORINEURAL HEARING LOSS

Congenital SNHL is inner ear hearing loss present at birth (may be hereditary or non-hereditary).

Hereditary defects can be classified as:
- Non-syndrome associated (65%):
    - Hearing impairment only.
    - Most inherited as an autosomal recessive trait.
- Syndrome associated (35%):
    - Hearing impairment is associated with other symptoms – the hearing loss is a feature of a syndrome e.g.:
    - Waardenburg syndrome.
    - CHARGE syndrome.
    - Treacher-Collins syndrome.
    - Alport syndrome.

See key syndrome features below

Non-hereditary defects involve direct damage to the developing cochlea that include intrauterine infections, medications or teratogens.
- Intrauterine infections (e.g., Toxoplasmosis, Rubella, CMV, Herpes Simplex, Syphilis).
- Medications (e.g., ototoxic drugs).
- Teratogens (e.g., alcohol, retinoic acid).

FACTORS RELATING TO INNER EAR DISEASE

Prematurity	Hypoxia
Craniofacial abnormality	Kernicterus
Ototoxic drugs	Neonatal sepsis
Intrauterine infections	Perinatal infections
Family history of childhood hearing impairment	NICU admission

Waardenburg Syndrome – White forelock and pale eyes with heterochromia.

CHARGE Syndrome stands for Coloboma, Heart defects, Atresia of the choanae, Retardation of Growth, Ear abnormalities.

Treacher-Collins Syndrome – Downward slanting eyes and small chin associated with facial bone maldevelopment.

Alport Syndrome – Renal abnormalities with oedema, haematuria, proteinuria and hypertension.

PRESBYCUSIS

Definition
- Age-related sensorineural hearing loss affecting persons over 50 years.

Epidemiology
- More common in men.
- More than half of adult population affected by age 75.

Aetiology
- Degeneration of hair cells, spiral ganglion cells and basilar membrane.

Clinical Presentation
- Progressive, symmetrical hearing loss at high frequencies.
- Poor speech recognition, especially with background noise.
- Tinnitus may be present.

Investigation
- Audiogram: Symmetrical SNHL that is more severe than normal age related hearing loss.

Treatment
- No specific medical or surgical treatment.
- Bilateral hearing aids if significant hearing loss.
- Auditory rehabilitation.

Presbycusis (Worsening with age)

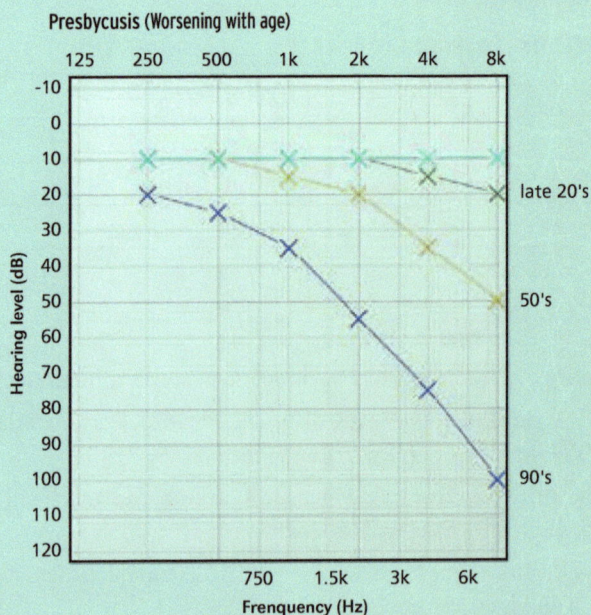

NOISE-INDUCED SENSORINEURAL HEARING LOSS

Definition
- Exposure to loud noise causing SNHL.

Classification
- Acute noise-induced hearing loss:
    - Exposure to high levels of noise lasting seconds to hours (e.g., music concerts, power tools).
    - Often reversible.
- Chronic noise-induced hearing loss:
    - Long term exposure to significant noise levels (e.g., workplace / machinery).
    - Irreversible hearing loss.

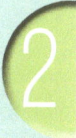

Pathophysiology
- Direct mechanical damage to the cochlea and metabolic injury due to overstimulation.

Clinical Presentation
- Acute: Sudden bilateral hearing loss, tinnitus.
- Chronic: Gradual hearing loss, loss of speech discrimination, tinnitus.

Investigation
- Audiogram: Initially a drop off at 4 kHz is characteristic and known as 'Boilermaker's notch'.

Treatment
- Hearing protection (e.g., ear muffs, ear plugs).
- If significant, consider hearing aids.

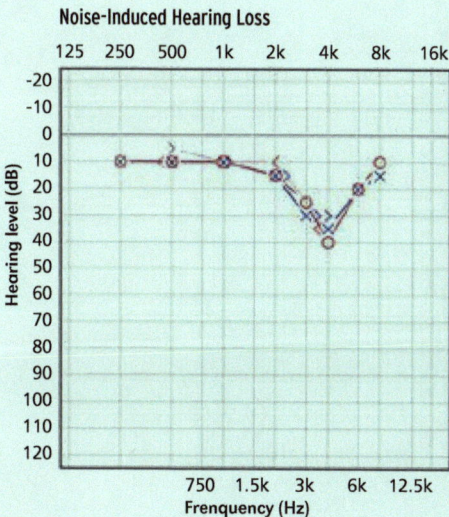

Noise-Induced Hearing Loss

SUDDEN SENSORINEURAL HEARING LOSS

Definition

- Sudden onset of SNHL (almost always unilateral).

Aetiology

- Cause unknown.
- Possible viral, vascular or autoimmune.

Clinical Presentation

- Sudden unilateral hearing loss.
- Tinnitus often present.
- May have vertigo.

Investigation

- Audiogram.
- MRI to exclude retrocochlear lesion.

Treatment

- No strong evidence for any therapy.
- First line of therapy is oral corticosteroids. If incomplete recovery then offer intratympanic steroid between weeks 2 to 6 after onset.

Prognosis

- Greater than 50% of patients show complete improvement.
- Worse prognosis when hearing loss is across all frequencies.

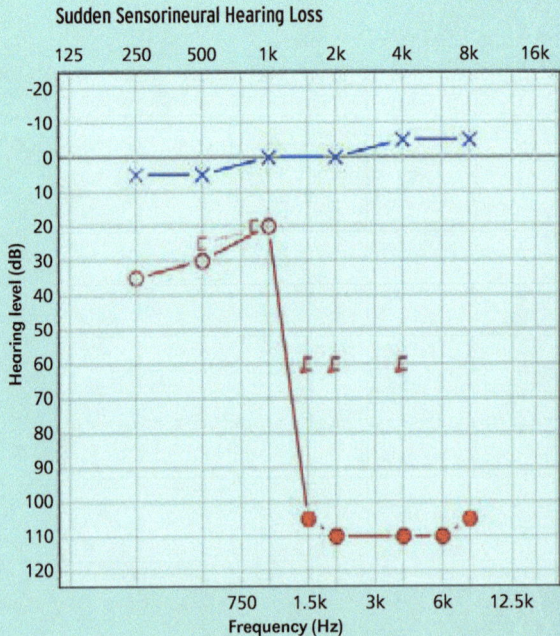

Sudden Sensorineural Hearing Loss

AUTOIMMUNE INNER EAR DISEASE

Definition
- An autoimmune disease leading to inner ear disease and hearing loss.

Aetiology
- Primary autoimmune disease arising in the inner ear.
- May be part of a systemic autoimmune disease (e.g., Wegeners granulomatosis – now renamed Granulomatosis with polyangiitis, Cogans syndrome, Rheumatoid arthritis, Systemic Lupus erythematosis).

Clinical Presentation
- Bilateral, asymmetrical SNHL that can be progressive or fluctuating.
- Vertigo and tinnitus may be present.

Investigation
- Autoimmune workup: ESR, ANA, Rheumatoid factor, Heat shock protein testing (HSP).

Treatment
- High dose corticosteroids for 2-3 weeks.
- Cytotoxic medications may be used if corticosteroids fail.

DRUG OTOTOXICITY

Definition
- A number of drugs cause toxic damage to the inner ear affecting hearing and/or vestibular function. The effects may not always be reversible.

Clinical Presentation
- Generally symmetrical hearing loss.
- Tinnitus may be present.

Treatment
- Discontinue ototoxic drug if possible.

OTOTOXIC DRUGS

Aminoglycosides	Streptomycin Gentamicin Tobramycin Amikacin Neomycin
Cytotoxic drugs	Cisplatin Bleomycin
Other	Loop Diuretics (Frusemide) Salicylates Quinine

VESTIBULAR DISORDERS

Vertigo is a symptom of illusion of movement of oneself or the environment, most commonly a spinning sensation.

Patients generally present with dizziness, so it is important to distinguish vertigo from other descriptions of dizziness such as presyncope and disequilibrium.

Vertigo can have a peripheral (inner ear) or a central (brainstem-cerebellum) aetiology.

CLINICAL FEATURES OF PERIPHERAL VS CENTRAL VERTIGO

	Peripheral	Central
Nystagmus	Unidirectional Horizontal or rotatory	Bidirectional Horizontal or vertical
Nausea and vomiting	Severe	Variable
Auditory symptoms	May be present	Absent
Neurological signs	Absent	Often present
Postural instability	Unidirectional instability, walking preserved	Severe, often falls when walking

BENIGN PAROXYSMAL POSITIONAL VERTIGO (BPPV)
Definition
- Intense, brief episodes of vertigo associated with changes in the position of the head.

Epidemiology
- More common in women.
- The posterior semicircular canal is mainly affected.

Aetiology
- Idiopathic.
- Head trauma.
- Viral infection.

Pathophysiology
- Due to loose calcium debris (otoliths) within the semicircular canals that are dislodged from their normal position.
  When the head changes position, these otoliths cause abnormal displacement of the endolymph in the affected semicircular canal resulting in a spinning sensation.

Clinical Presentation
- Recurrent episodes of vertigo lasting less than a minute.
- Provoked by certain head movements (e.g., rolling over in bed).
- May be associated with nausea and vomiting.

Diagnosis
- History.
- The Dix-Hallpike Test: With the patient seated upright, turn the head 45 degrees to one side. Next, quickly lie the patient back with the head hanging over the edge of the bed. The test is positive if this provokes nystagmus and vertigo. Repeat this test with the head turned to the other side. In BPPV the nystagmus and vertigo will usually fatigue with repetition and may completely settle after several repeats of the manoeuvre.

Treatment
- Reassure patient the vertigo will generally resolve spontaneously over days to weeks.
- Particle repositioning manoeuvres: Epley Manoeuvre.
- Surgery may be indicated in refractory BPPV.

The Dix-Hallpike Test

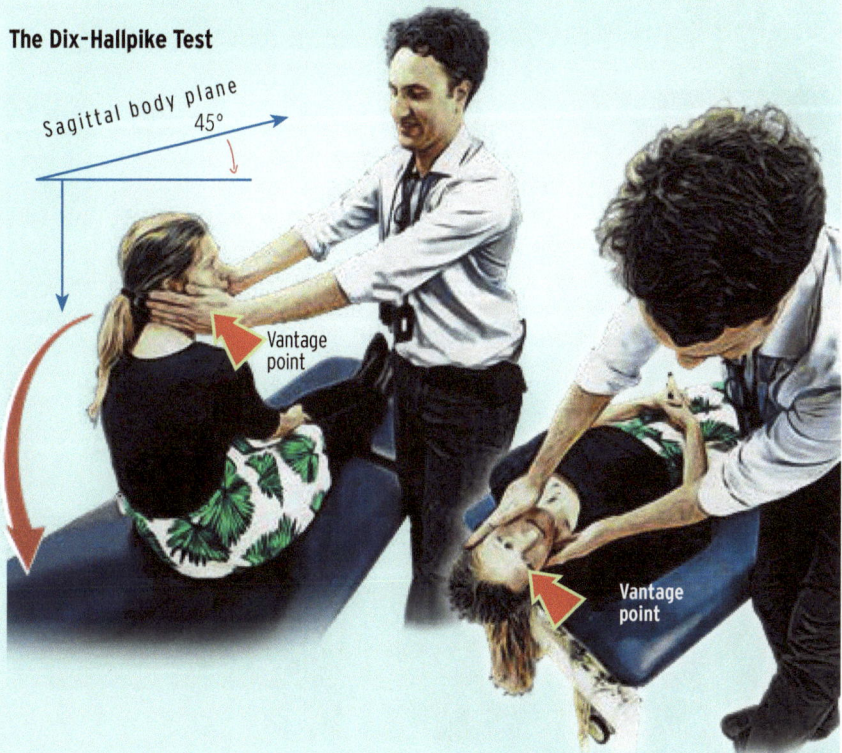

Sagittal body plane 45°

Vantage point

Vantage point

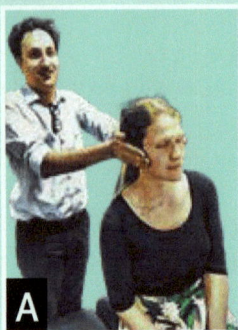

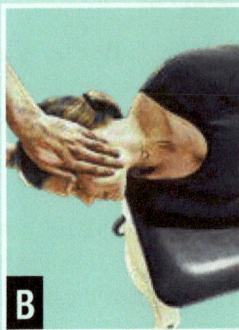

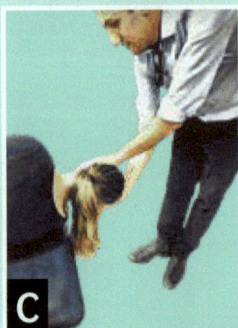

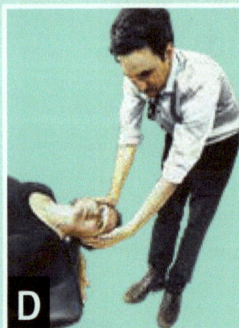

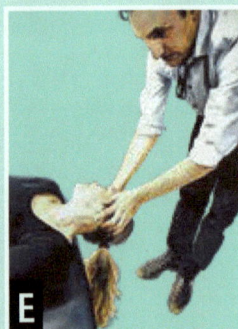

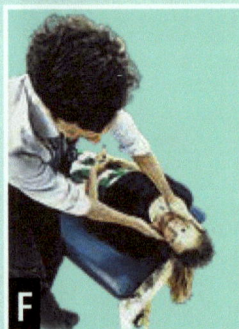

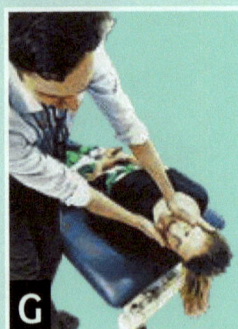

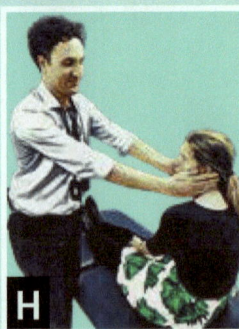

Epley Manoeuvre:

The first steps (A-C) is the Dix-Hallpike Test. In this example the right side is affected.

The head is next rotated 90 degrees to the left (D) and held in this position for 30 seconds.

The patient next rolls their whole body to the left (E) and holds this position for a further 30 seconds.

Lastly, the patient sits up (H) and should experience symptom relief.

VESTIBULAR NEURITIS

Definition
- Inflammation of the inner ear and/or vestibulocochlear nerve.

Epidemiology
- More common in middle-aged adults.

Aetiology
- Not completely understood.
- Disease appears two weeks after a viral URTI in less than half of the patients.

Clinical Presentation
- Sudden onset of severe vertigo.
- Associated with nausea, vomiting and gait instability.
- Symptoms generally resolve in a few days, although residual imbalance may persist for months.

Investigation
- Positive head impulse test.
- CT scan / MRI.

Treatment
- In the acute phase:
  - Bed rest.
  - Corticosteroids.
  - Antivertiginous drugs (e.g., Prochlorperazine) for the first 48 hours.
- Vestibular rehabilitation for patients with residual imbalance.

Head Impulse Test

Normal VOR (Vestibular ocular reflex)

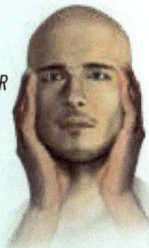

Patient focussed on examiner's nose

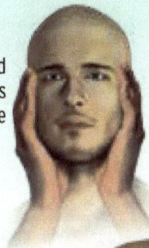

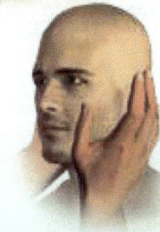

After sharp turn to patient's right, patient remains focussed on examiner's nose

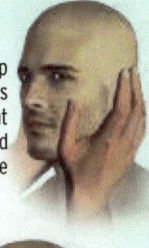

Abnormal VOR

Patient focussed on examiner's nose

Corrective saccades

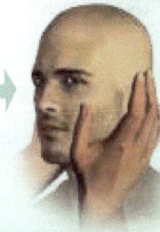

MENIERE'S DISEASE

Definition
- An inner ear disorder characterised by a combination of hearing loss, buzzing tinnitus, pressure sensation with vertigo.

Epidemiology
- Rare disorder.
- Symptom onset between the third and fifth decade of life.
- Rarely affects bilateral ears.

Aetiology
- Poorly understood.
- Most cases are idiopathic.

Pathophysiology
- Distortion of the membranous labyrinth due to endolymph accumulation (endolymphatic hydrops).

Risk factors
- Family history.

Clinical Presentation
- Attacks of vertigo lasting from minutes to hours. May be associated with nausea and vomiting.
- Fluctuating sensorineural hearing loss. Progresses over time, initially affecting lower frequencies.
- Tinnitus.
- May have sudden falls without loss of consciousness (Tumarkin crisis/drop attack) late in the disease course, although rare.

Diagnosis
- Clinical diagnosis.

Treatment
- Lifestyle changes: Avoid high salt intake, caffeine, alcohol, nicotine.
- Medical management includes: Antivertiginous drugs, anti-emetics. Thiazide diuretics and betahistine.
- For severe symptoms, despite maximal medical management, consider:
  - Transtympanic gentamicin.
  - Vestibular neurectomy.
  - Labyrinthectomy.
  - Endolymphatic sac decompression.

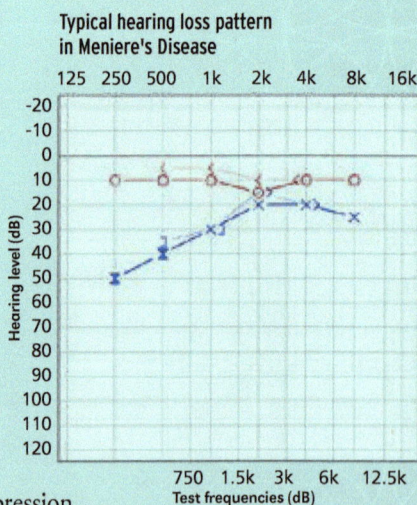

Typical hearing loss pattern in Meniere's Disease

ACOUSTIC NEUROMA

Definition
- Benign tumour of the Schwann cells of the vestibulocochlear nerve.

Epidemiology
- Makes up the majority of tumours of the cerebellopontine angle.
- Majority of tumours are unilateral.

Clinical Presentation
- Unilateral sensorineural hearing loss and tinnitus.
- Later symptoms include disequilibrium, vertigo and facial hypoesthesia.
- Extension to the brainstem can lead to hydrocephalus and death.

Investigation
- Weber and Rinne tests.
- Audiometry.
- CT scan / MRI.

Treatment
- Small tumours, slowly progressive tumours or tumours in the elderly may undergo observation with regular follow up.
- Large tumours or younger patients may require surgery or radiotherapy.

Cerebellar meningioma, adjacent to internal auditory canal – compare with Acoustic neuroma

Acoustic neuroma (left)

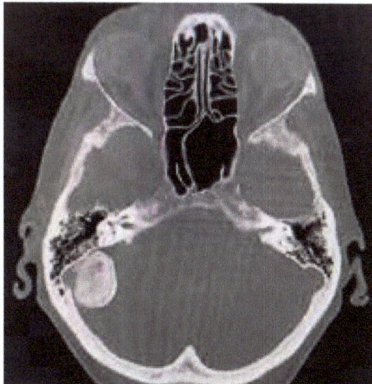

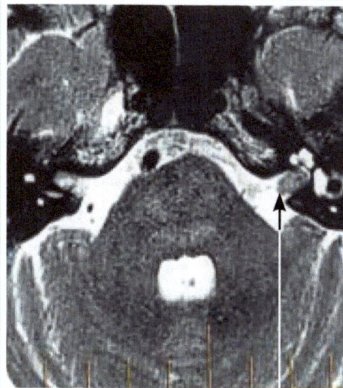

Acoustic neuroma in internal auditory canal

	Time course	Auditory symptoms	Neurological symptoms	Diagnostic features
Benign Paroxysmal Positional Vertigo	Recurrent, lasting seconds	None	None	Positive Dix-Hallpike Test
Vestibular Neuritis	Single episode, lasting days	None	Unsteady towards the side of the lesion	Abnormal head impulse test
Meniere's Disease	Recurrent, lasting minutes to hours	Fluctuating SNHL and tinnitus	None	Unilateral low frequency SNHL
Acoustic Neuroma	Chronic, late stage of disease	Unilateral hearing loss and tinnitus	Disequilibrium and facial hypaesthesia	

A PRACTICAL APPROACH TO VERTIGO

Modified from J. Kanagalingam B.M.J. March 2005

The common complaint of dizziness means different things to different patients.

To differentiate the common divisions ask:

- Does the room spin (vertigo)?
- Do you feel unsteady (dysequilibrium)?
- Do you feel as if you will faint (presyncope)?
- Do you feel light-headed?

Vertigo is an illusion of movement. When associated with nausea and vomiting, it indicates a peripheral cause (related to the ear) as opposed to central (brain related).

Dysequilibrium occurs when the ears and eyes do not provide enough information to the brain about the body's position e.g., peripheral neuropathy, eye disease or peripheral vestibular disorders.

Presyncope is caused by cardiovascular disorders reducing cerebral perfusion.

Light-headedness is hard to diagnose due to being non-specific but results from anxiety, panic attacks and hyperventilation.

Examination includes:

- Cranial nerves. Especially look for papilloedema cranial nerve II.
- Eye movements III, IV, VI.
- Corneal reflex V.
- Facial movements VII.

Nystagmus is common in acute vertigo.
Check cerebellar function:

- Past pointing.
- Dysdiadochokinesia.
- Vibration sense on ankle for neuropathy.
- Otoscopy – helpful when hearing loss or pain.
- Dix-Hallpike Test for BPPV.

Diagnosis:

- Helped by description of vertigo.
- The precipitants and time course.
- The frequency and duration.
- Rarely vertigo from brainstem CVA, intracranial lesions or migraine.

The following are 'Red Flag' features that indicate a non-vestibular that is a central cause.

> *Key Point:* Persistent, worsening vertigo or dysequillibrium. Atypical 'non-peripheral' vertigo with vertical nystagmus with vertical movement, severe headache, diplopia, cranial nerve palsies, dysarthria, ataxia, cerebellar signs and papilloedema.

What to do:

Explain the vertigo.
Medication.
Epley Manoeuvre.
Cawthorne-Cooksey excersises.
Refer if recurring / persistent / vertigo with peripheral vestibular features or abnormal otoscopy.

EVALUATION OF TINNITUS

Tinnitus is a perception of sound in the absence of an external stimuli. The sound is often described as a ringing or buzzing in the ears. It can be continuous or intermittent, pulsatile or non-pulsatile.

Tinnitus is a nonspecific symptom with a broad list of causes:

Auditory
- Presbycusis.
- Ototoxic medications.
- Acoustic neuroma.
- Otosclerosis.
- Meniere's Disease.
- Trauma (barotrauma, head injuries).

Vascular
- Arteriovenous malformation.
- Paraganglioma.
- Arterial bruits and venous hums.

Other
- Metabolic disease.
- Eustachian tube dysfunction.
- TMJ dysfunction.

Investigation
- Audiogram.
- Consider CT scan / MRI if suspected retrocochlear lesion.
- Metabolic workup (thyroid function tests, lipid profile).

SURGERY FOR HEARING IMPROVEMENT

Clearance of disease affecting hearing has been discussed above e.g., cholesteatomas.

However, surgical improvement in hearing can be brought about by various procedures e.g., ossicular chain reconstruction or stapes surgery to allow transmission of vibration through a thickened/fixed stapes bone.

In some situations (e.g., middle ear disease), the ear canal is by-passed by a bone anchored hearing aid (BAHA) where electro-magnetic vibrations pass through the scalp skin to an implanted device which transmits the vibrations to the cochleas of both ears.

In situations where cochlea function has been damaged, the remaining neural structures can be helped by cochlea implantation which is a major advance in patient management.

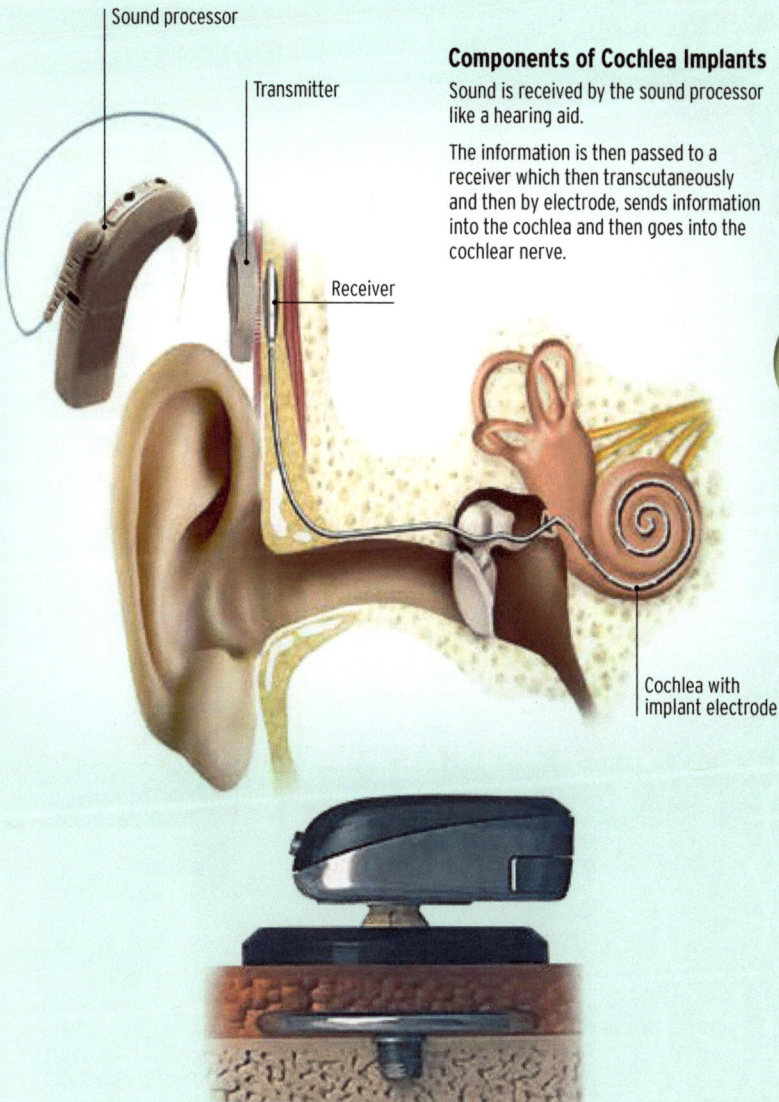

Sound processor

Transmitter

Receiver

Components of Cochlea Implants

Sound is received by the sound processor like a hearing aid.

The information is then passed to a receiver which then transcutaneously and then by electrode, sends information into the cochlea and then goes into the cochlear nerve.

Cochlea with implant electrode

BAHA: Bone Anchored Hearing Aid.
Metal disc screwed into skull bone and hearing aid attached to skin by magnetism and transmits vibration through skin to the bone which takes the vibrations to both cochleae.

CHAPTER 3

Rhinology

This is the study of the Rhino (nose). It has both external and internal components and posteriorly joins the naso pharynx. Not only does it filter, warm and humidify air to aid oxygen transfer but it is the structure for smell and is the pathway of drainage from the sinuses and eyes.

Structures of the Nose

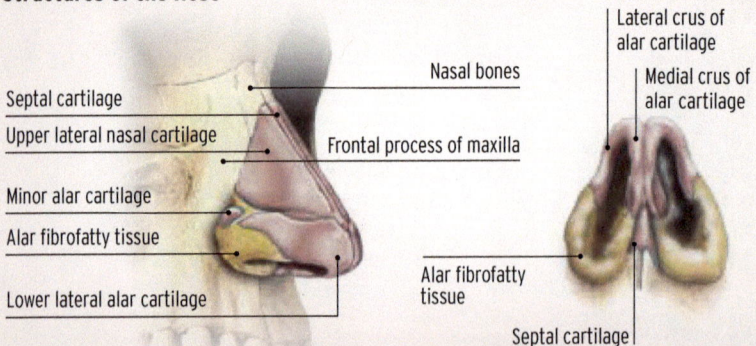

Septal cartilage
Upper lateral nasal cartilage
Minor alar cartilage
Alar fibrofatty tissue
Lower lateral alar cartilage

Nasal bones
Frontal process of maxilla

Lateral crus of alar cartilage
Medial crus of alar cartilage
Alar fibrofatty tissue
Septal cartilage

ANATOMY OF THE NOSE AND SINUSES

The nose is made up of a framework of bone and cartilage and is divided into left and right chambers by a nasal septum. The lateral walls of the nasal cavity have three bony projections that project into the nasal cavity which are called the superior, middle and inferior turbinates.

The nose serves as an initial conduit for the passage of air into the respiratory tract. Airflow through the nose is more efficient in gas exchange and requires less energy than mouth breathing. Other important functions of the nose include warming and humidifying the air and for olfaction and also forms part of the defence against infections.

The paranasal sinuses are air-filled cavities, lined with mucosa, that communicate directly with the nasal cavity. There are four pairs of paranasal sinuses – the frontal, maxillary, ethmoidal and sphenoidal sinuses.

Lateral Wall of Nose

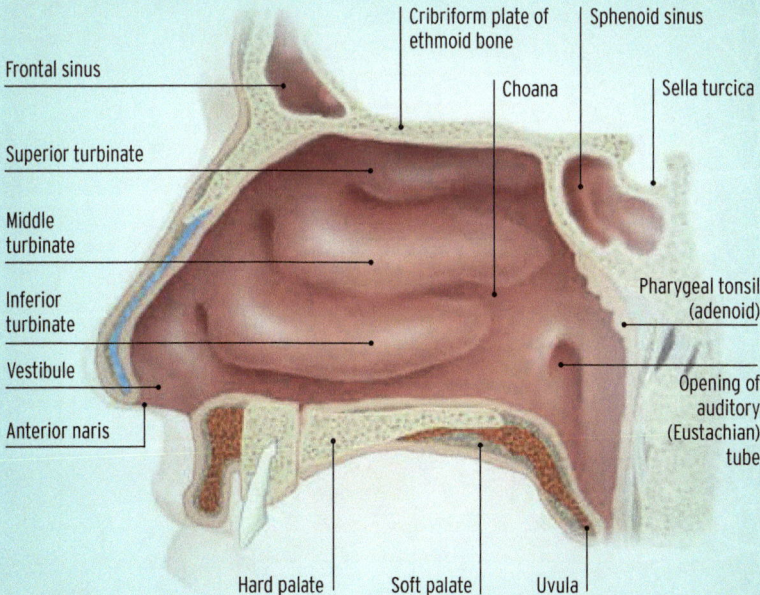

Frontal sinus

Cribriform plate of ethmoid bone

Sphenoid sinus

Choana

Sella turcica

Superior turbinate

Middle turbinate

Inferior turbinate

Pharygeal tonsil (adenoid)

Vestibule

Opening of auditory (Eustachian) tube

Anterior naris

Hard palate

Soft palate

Uvula

RHINITIS

Definition
- Inflammation of the nasal cavity mucosa.

Classification
- Nonallergic rhinitis.
- Allergic rhinitis.

1. NONALLERGIC RHINITIS
Typically presents with clear rhinorrhoea and nasal obstruction.
It is uncommon to present with sneezing or itchy/watery eyes. See table for the types of nonallergic rhinitis.

Treatment
- Nonsurgical measures: Irritant avoidance, saline irrigation, topical steroids, adrenergic agents and anticholinergic agents.
- Surgical measures: Septoplasty and turbinate surgery.

Allergic Rhinitis	Nonallergic Rhinitis
• Seasonal • Perennial	• Viral • Bacterial rhinosinusitis • Vasomotor rhinitis • Occupational rhinitis • Rhinitis medicamentosa • Rhinitis of pregnancy • Hypothyroidism • Medications (e.g., OCP) • Granulomatous rhinitis • Atrophic rhinitis • Gustatory rhinitis

2. ALLERGIC RHINITIS

Definition
- Allergic rhinitis is inflammation of the nasal mucosa caused by an IgE-mediated hypersensitivity reaction to foreign allergens.

Classification
- Seasonal.
- Perennial.

Epidemiology
- Incidence of onset is greatest in adolescence, however, can occur at any age.

Aetiology

- May be influenced by: Genetic susceptibility, environmental factors, exposure to allergens or passive exposure to smoke.

Pathophysiology

- In patients with a predisposition, sensitisation to a specific allergen (generally airborne) induces IgE antibody production.
- On subsequent exposure, the attachment of the specific antigen to the IgE antibodies provokes an inflammatory response leading to the clinical presentation.

Clinical Presentation

- Seasonal Allergic Rhinitis:
    - Symptoms occur or are increased during certain seasons.
    - Usually due to pollen.
    - Watery rhinorrhoea, red and watery eyes, sneezing, nasal congestion and itching of the nose, eyes, ears and throat.
    - Nasal examination: Wet, swollen mucosa and bluish, pale turbinates.
- Perennial Allergic Rhinitis:
    - Symptoms are constant with little seasonal variation.
    - Usually due to dust mites and animal dander.
    - Nasal congestion and postnasal drip. Rhinorrhoea, eye symptoms and sneezing are less common.
    - Nasal examination: Normal.

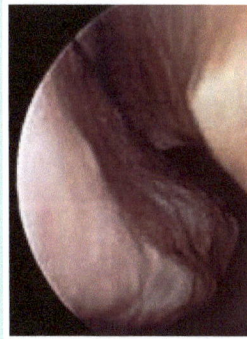

Investigations

- Allergy history.
- Allergy testing, skin testing and in vitro testing.

Anterior view into right nasal cavity. Inferior turbinate inferiorly and deviated septum.

Treatment

- Avoidance of allergens and environmental controls.
- Pharmacotherapy:
    - Antihistamines.
    - Intranasal corticosteroids.
    - Nasal decongestants.
    - Systemic corticosteroids.
    - Intranasal anticholinergics.
    - Intranasal cromolyn.
    - Leukotriene inhibitors.
- Immunotherapy.
- Surgical: Turbinate reduction.

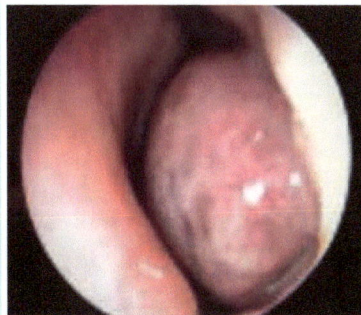

Enlarged (allergic) inferior turbinate on the right. Note: Curvature of the septum on the left.

RHINOSINUSITIS

Definition
- Rhinosinusitis is a group of disorders characterised by inflammation of the nasal cavity and paranasal sinuses.

Classification
- Acute rhinosinusitis.
- Chronic rhinosinusitis.

1. ACUTE RHINOSINUSITIS

Definition
- Inflammation of the paranasal sinuses lasting less than 4 weeks.

Epidemiology
- Most commonly affects the maxillary sinus in adults.
- Majority of cases are viral infections.
- Bacterial infections are less common.

Aetiology
- Causative agents:
  - Viral: Rhinovirus, influenza virus, parainfluenza virus.
  - Bacterial: S. pneumoniae; H. influenzae; M. catarrhalis.

Pathophysiology
- Results from the spread of inflammation of the nasal cavity into the paranasal sinuses.

Risk factors
- Older age.
- Smoking.
- Allergies.
- Dental disease.

Clinical Presentation
- Nasal congestion/obstruction, rhinorrhoea, facial pain/pressure.
- Fever, anosmia/hyposmia, headache, ear pain/pressure, halitosis, fatigue, dental pain.
- Viral causes have complete or partial improvement by day 7 to 10.
- Bacterial causes generally have symptoms persisting beyond 10 days and of a greater severity.

Investigation
- Rhinoscopy: Mucosal oedema, rhinorrhoea or purulent discharge.
- Swab of nasal mucosa/discharge.
- CT scan/MRI: Consider when complications present.

Treatment
- Symptomatic management: Analgesia, saline irrigation, intranasal corticosteroids.
- Consider antibiotics if bacterial cause is implicated (clinically or positive swab result).

COMPLICATIONS

Orbital	Intracranial	Bone
Periorbital cellulitis	Meningitis	Osteitis of the sinus bones
Orbital cellulitis	Intracranial abscess	
Subperiosteal abscess	Epidural abscess	

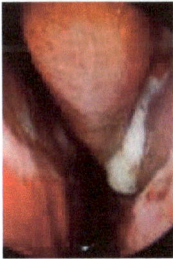

Pus in the middle meatus sitting beside the middle turbinate

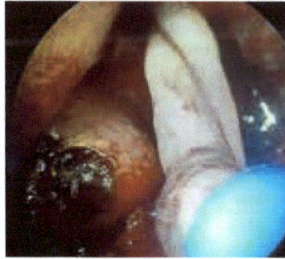

Muco pus being suctioned from the frontal sinus

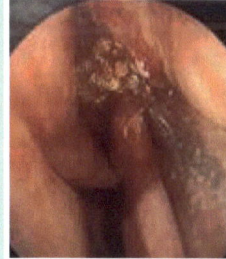

Fungus being suctioned from the maxillary sinus

Chronic Sinusitis – double density in maxillary sinus indicating fungus

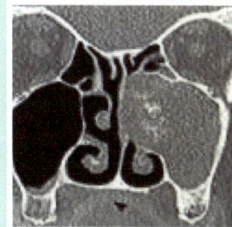

2. CHRONIC RHINOSINUSITIS

Definition
- Inflammation of the paranasal sinuses lasting greater than 12 weeks.

Classification
- Chronic rhinosinusitis without nasal polyps.
- Chronic rhinosinusitis with nasal polyps.
- Allergic fungal rhinosinusitis.

Epidemiology
- Occurs in both children and adults, although more commonly diagnosed in middle-aged adults.
- Large economic burden and impact on quality of life.

Aetiology

- Anatomic abnormalities (e.g., septal deviation).
- Allergic rhinitis.
- Systemic disorders (polyangitis and granulomatosis) was called Wegener's Disease.
- Chronic exposure to irritants.
- Immunocompromised states.
- Mucociliary clearance defects (e.g., cystic fibrosis).

Pathophysiology

- Obstruction of the ostiomeatal complex leading to impairment of sinus drainage.

Clinical Presentation

- Chronic nasal congestion/obstruction, rhinorrhoea, facial pain/pressure.
- Fever, anosmia/hyposmia, headache, ear pain/pressure, halitosis, fatigue, dental pain.

Investigation

- Rhinoscopy/endoscopy: Nasal septum, turbinates and ostiomeatal complex.
- CT scan.
- Allergy testing.

NASAL POLYPS

- May be benign or malignant. Commonly related to allergy and infection.

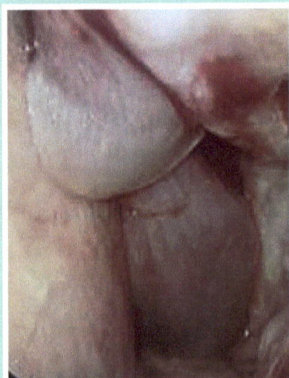

Nasal polyps within the nose

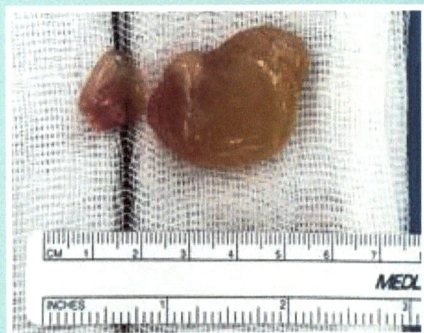

Nasal polyps at surgery

Key Point: Regard the unilateral polyp to be malignant until proven otherwise.

Treatment

- Goal is to reduce symptoms.
- Includes combinations of saline washes, intranasal and oral corticosteroids and antibiotics. Many patients with chronic rhinosinusitis show a type 2 inflammatory response. Specific drugs are becoming available for selected patients. These so called biologics include the type 2 targeting agents such as anti-IgE.
- Surgery if medical management fails: Functional Endoscopic Sinus Surgery (FESS).

Complications

- Same as for acute rhinosinusitis.

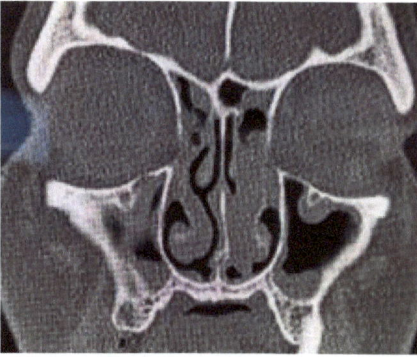

Polyp in left nasal cavity

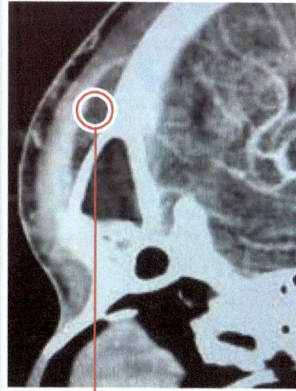

Potts puffy tumour – abscess over the frontal bone

Potts Puffy Tumour

A complication of frontal sinusitis where a subperiosteal abscess forms.

EPISTAXIS

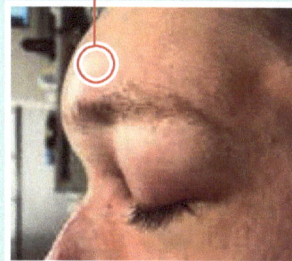

Potts puffy tumour

Definition

- Bleeding from the nose.

Epidemiology

- Common but infrequently requiring medical attention.
- Anterior bleeds more common than posterior bleeds – most arising from Kiesselbach's plexus.

Aetiology

- Local:
    - Digital trauma.
    - Facial trauma.
    - Foreign body.

- Septal perforations (chronic intranasal drug use and trauma).
- Mucosal dryness.
- Rhinitis.
- Neoplasia.
- Idiopathic.
- Systemic diseases (e.g., coagulopathies, platelet disorders, hypertension).

Investigation
- Bloods: FBC, coagulation studies and group and hold (if indicated).
- Anterior rhinoscopy.
- Endoscopic examination.

Treatment
- ABC.

> ***Key Point:*** If no bleeding point can be found in a patient over 60, get CT scan of the sinuses.

- Conservative measures:
  - Spray nasal cavity with oxymetazoline.
  - Patient to pinch alae against the nasal septum.
- Local measures if above fails:
  - Locate the source of bleeding with rhinoscopy and headlight.
  - Cautery (e.g., silver nitrate sticks/thermal cautery).
  - Anterior nasal packing (tampons, balloons).
- If bleeding persists, likely a posterior bleed:
  - Balloon catheter (e.g., Rapid Rhino Balloon).
- Endoscopic ligation or embolisation if bleeding persists.

Epistaxis Treatment Summary
This may be trivial or catastrophic. Common causes are trauma, hypertension and anticoagulants/blood disorders.
- Bleeding requires examination with headlight and specula or endoscope.
- Trivial bleeds may be treated with chemical or thermal cautery or pressure. May be helped by antibiotic ointment and antibiotic and/or vaso constricting agents.
- Major bleeds may preclude good visualisation and generalised treatment is required.
  - Resuscitate the patient – Blood/IV fluids.
  - Tranexamic acid.
  - Pressure to the bleeding site e.g., Rapid Rhino Balloon or Foley catheter or similar.
  - Control blood pressure.
  - Avoid blood thinning agents.

Complications
- Consider antibiotics for prolonged nasal packing due to the risk of developing toxic shock syndrome.

Blood Supply to Nasal Septum

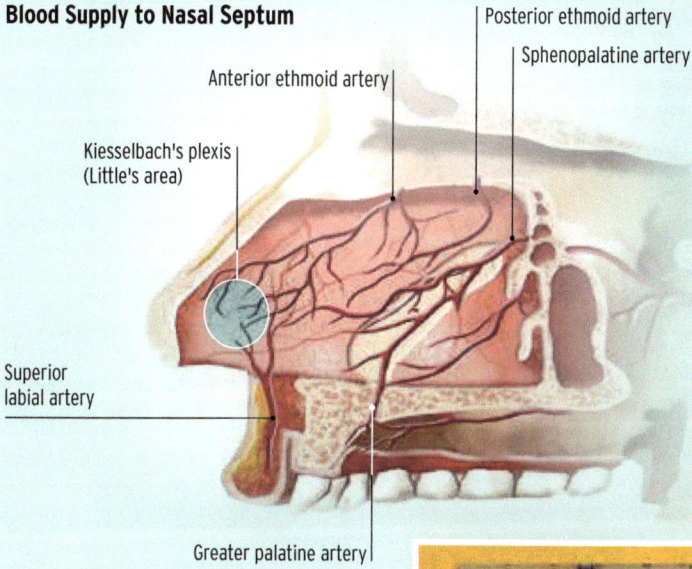

- Posterior ethmoid artery
- Sphenopalatine artery
- Anterior ethmoid artery
- Kiesselbach's plexis (Little's area)
- Superior labial artery
- Greater palatine artery

Rapid Rhino Balloon for epistoxis. Wet the gel coating for gentle insertion, then inflate.

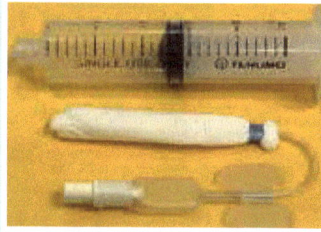

Endoscopic DCR (Dacryocystorhinostomy)

This procedure involves incision of the lacrimal sac accessed lateral to the nasal middle turbinate.

Incision and drainage of the sac allows relief of blockage and is the treatment for epiphora and dacryocystitis.

Silicone tubing may be left in place for some weeks to help maintain patency.

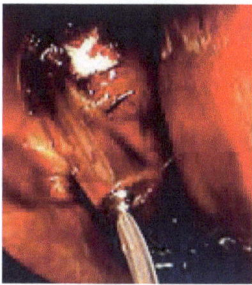

Tubing in lacrimal system following DCR

The Lacrimal System

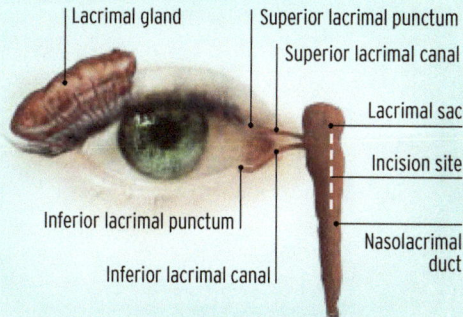

- Lacrimal gland
- Superior lacrimal punctum
- Superior lacrimal canal
- Lacrimal sac
- Incision site
- Inferior lacrimal punctum
- Inferior lacrimal canal
- Nasolacrimal duct

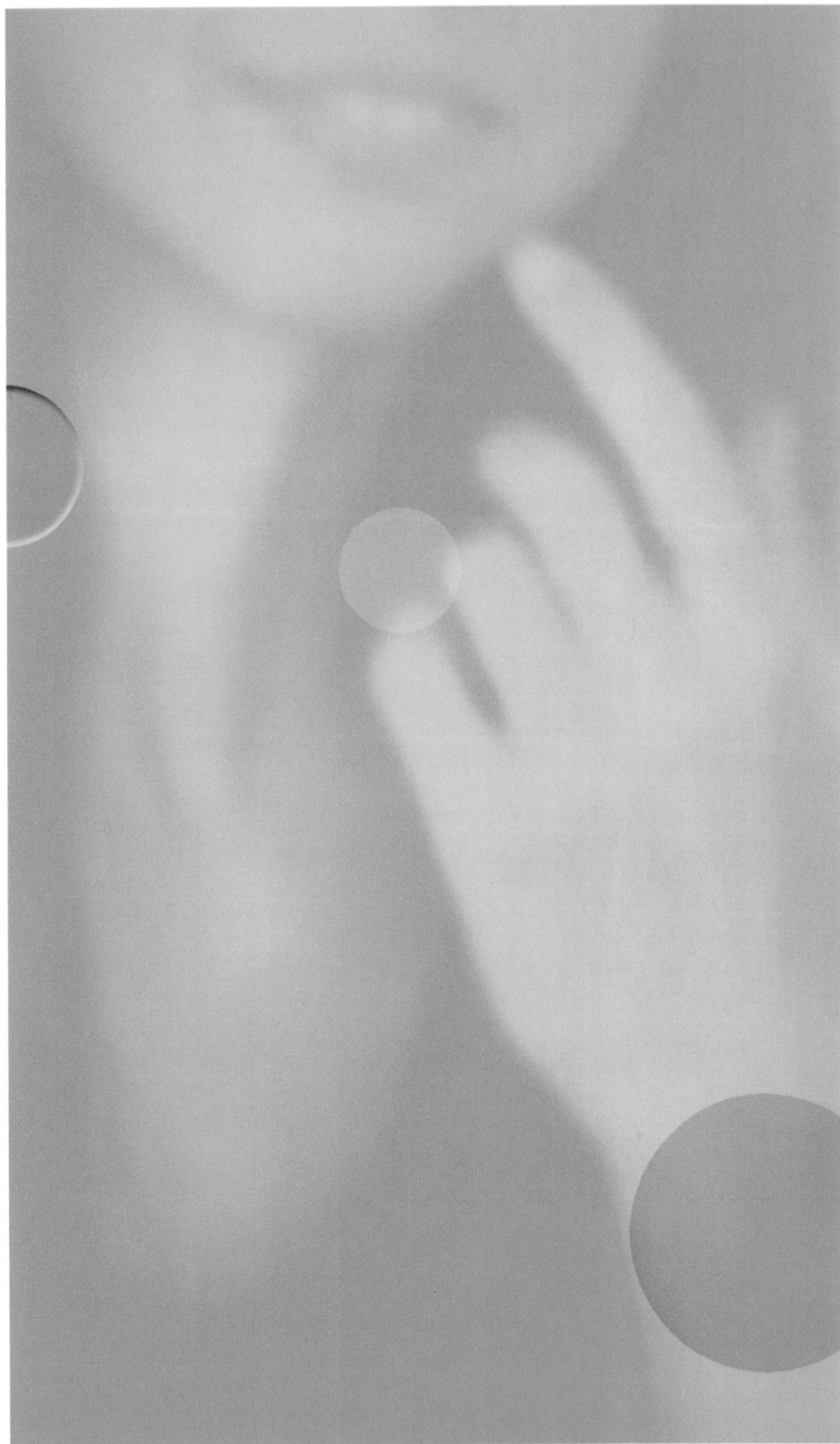

CHAPTER 4

Laryngology

This is the study of the larynx (voice box).
Voice production is the commonly identified function but protection
of the lungs from food and fluid entry is also a key function.

ANATOMY/PHYSIOLOGY

The larynx (voice box) is found central in the neck and lies between the oropharynx and the trachea. The larynx is made up of a cartilaginous skeleton and extrinsic and intrinsic muscles. It also houses the vocal folds. The extrinsic muscles of the neck are responsible for the positioning of the entire larynx in the neck. The intrinsic muscles are responsible for the movement of the vocal folds.

The larynx is involved in **phonation, respiration, cough and swallowing.** During expiration, the vocal folds are brought close together and oscillate generating sound. The pitch of the sound can be manipulated by changing the length and tension of the vocal folds. These sounds resonate into the pharynx and nose and are articulated into speech.

Swallowing: Inversion of the epiglottis and laryngeal elevation prevents food from entering the larynx. The vocal folds also close to prevent aspiration and a cough reflex is induced if the vocal folds are stimulated. These mechanisms ensure protection of the airway during swallowing.

Relations of the Pharynx and Larynx

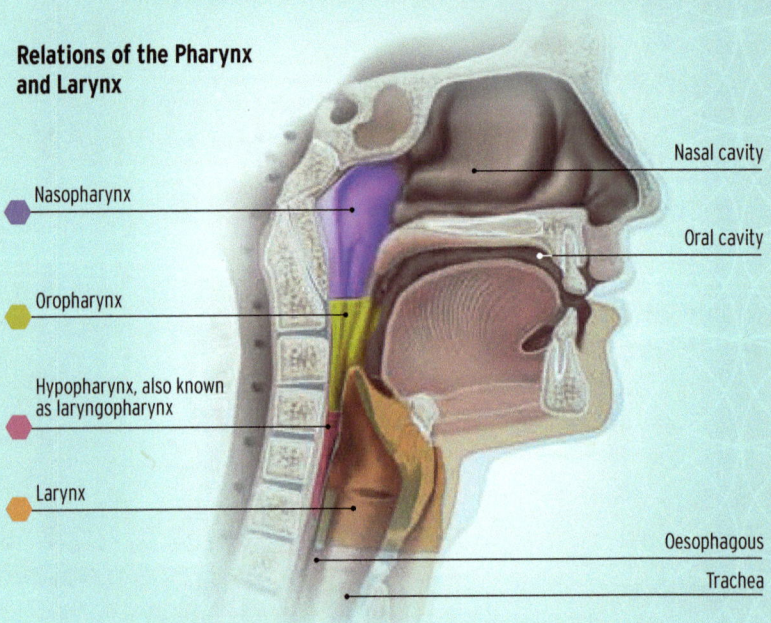

Nasal cavity

Nasopharynx

Oral cavity

Oropharynx

Hypopharynx, also known as laryngopharynx

Larynx

Oesophagous

Trachea

Anatomy of the Larynx

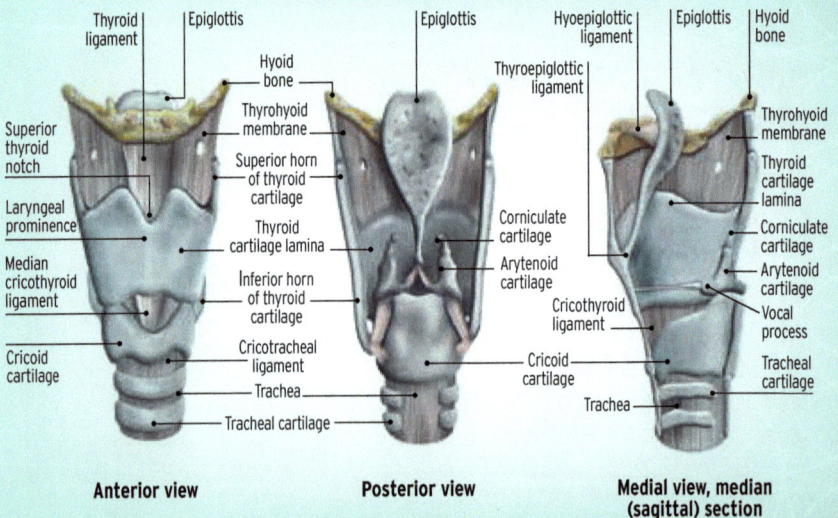

Thyroid ligament | Epiglottis

Hyoid bone

Thyrohyoid membrane

Superior horn of thyroid cartilage

Superior thyroid notch

Laryngeal prominence

Thyroid cartilage lamina

Median cricothyroid ligament

Inferior horn of thyroid cartilage

Cricoid cartilage

Cricotracheal ligament

Trachea

Tracheal cartilage

Anterior view

Epiglottis

Thyroepiglottic ligament

Corniculate cartilage

Arytenoid cartilage

Cricoid cartilage

Trachea

Posterior view

Hyoepiglottic ligament | Epiglottis | Hyoid bone

Thyrohyoid membrane

Thyroid cartilage lamina

Corniculate cartilage

Arytenoid cartilage

Cricothyroid ligament

Vocal process

Tracheal cartilage

Medial view, median (sagittal) section

View of Larynx at Endoscopy and Intubation

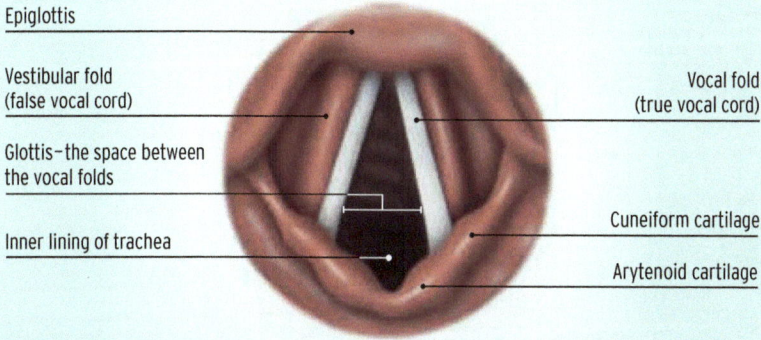

Epiglottis

Vestibular fold
(false vocal cord)

Vocal fold
(true vocal cord)

Glottis—the space between
the vocal folds

Cuneiform cartilage

Inner lining of trachea

Arytenoid cartilage

ACUTE LARYNGITIS

Definition
- Inflammation of the laryngeal mucosa lasting less than 2 weeks.

Aetiology
- Causative agents: Viral (influenza), bacterial (S. pneumoniae, H. influenzae, M. catarrhalis).

Pathophysiology
- Generally, an URTI descending to involve the larynx.
- Acute vocal strain can also result in submucosal trauma and vocal fold oedema.

Clinical Presentation
- Hoarseness.
- If URTI present: Rhinorrhoea, cough and sore throat.
- Dyspnoea if severe mucosal swelling.

Investigation
- Endoscopy: Vocal folds will be erythematous and oedematous with normal mobility.

Treatment
- Self-limiting course.
- Voice rest and inhalation therapy.
- Irritants should be avoided (e.g., cigarette smoke).
- Antibiotics if a concurrent bacterial infection.

Acute Laryngitis

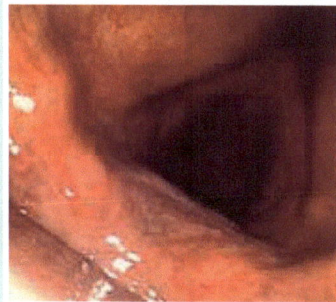

Erythema throughout the larynx –
similar appearance to chronic laryngitis

4

CHRONIC LARYNGITIS

Definition
- Inflammation of the laryngeal mucosa lasting more than 2 weeks.

Epidemiology
- More common in smokers.
- More common in elderly men.

Aetiology
- Chronic inhaled irritants (e.g., smoking).
- Chronic vocal overuse.
- Chronic rhinosinusitis.
- Gastro-oesophageal reflux disease.

Pathophysiology
- The irritants cause the epithelium to thicken and cause submucosal oedema.

Clinical Presentation
- Hoarseness.
- Dry cough, frequent throat clearing.

Investigation
- NPE (Nasopharyngeal Endoscopy): Vocal folds will be erythematous, thickened and ulcerated with normal mobility.

Treatment
- Remove the causative irritant.
- Inhalation therapy and mucolytics.
- Acute exacerbations treated with antibiotics and corticosteroids.
- Treat any related disorders.

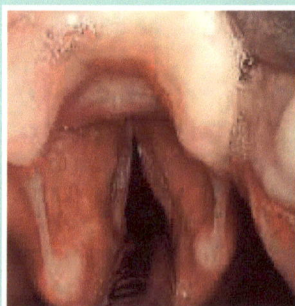

Chronic laryngitis

Key Point: Chronic laryngitis (hoarseness) cannot be clinically distinguished from early stage laryngeal cancer. Any persistent form of laryngitis requires fibre-optic examination for a specific diagnosis.

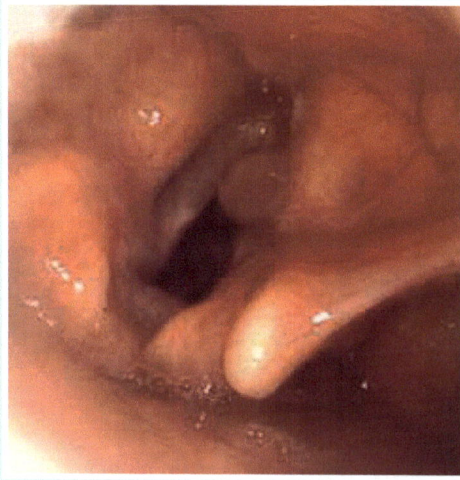

Vocal cord polyp

VOCAL FOLD POLYPS

Definition
- Benign fluid-filled collection on the vocal folds.

Epidemiology
- More common in males and adults.
- Mostly unilateral but can be bilateral.

Aetiology
- Vocal overuse.
- Chronic inflammation.

Pathophysiology
- Capillary damage in the subepithelial space.

Clinical Presentation
- Hoarseness, aphonia, cough.

Investigation
- NPE: Pedunculated or sessile polyp on vocal fold.

Treatment
- Microsurgical removal.
- Voice therapy.

LARYNGEAL PAPILLOMATOSIS

Definition
- HPV (Human Papilloma Virus) infection causing benign growths (papillomas) in the airway, including the vocal folds.

Epidemiology
- Most common laryngeal tumour in children.

Aetiology
- Causative agents: HPV, most notably type 6 and 11.

Clinical Presentation
- Hoarseness.
- Inspiratory stridor.
- Continued growth may cause life threatening airway obstruction.

Investigation
- NPE: Multiple wart-like lesions covering the glottis and supraglottis.

Treatment
- Microlaryngeal surgery – laser therapy.
- Interferon, acyclovir, photodynamic therapy are a few therapies under investigation.

Complications
- Potential for malignant transformation (especially HPV 16 and 18 subtypes).

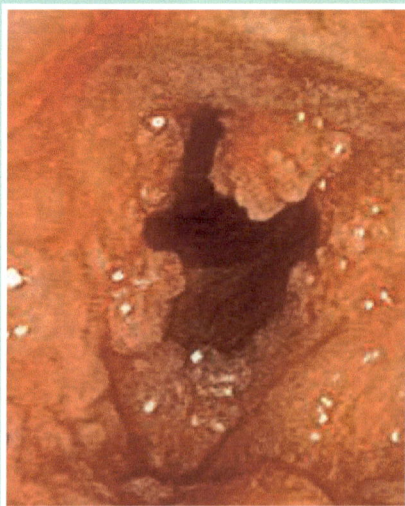

Laryngeal papilloma of the vocal cords

VOCAL FOLD NODULES

Definition
- Thickening or callus formation on the vocal folds.

Epidemiology
- Common in singers, children, teachers and professional speakers.
- More common in woman.

Aetiology
- Chronic vocal fold irritation through vocal abuse, smoking and reflux.

Clinical Presentation
- Hoarseness.
- Diplophonia and globus sensation.

Investigation
- NPE: Bilateral nodules seen at the junction of the anterior and middle thirds of the vocal fold (point of maximum vibration).

Treatment
- Voice rest.
- Avoid causal irritants.
- Speech therapy.
- Surgery rarely indicated.

4

Bilateral vocal nodules

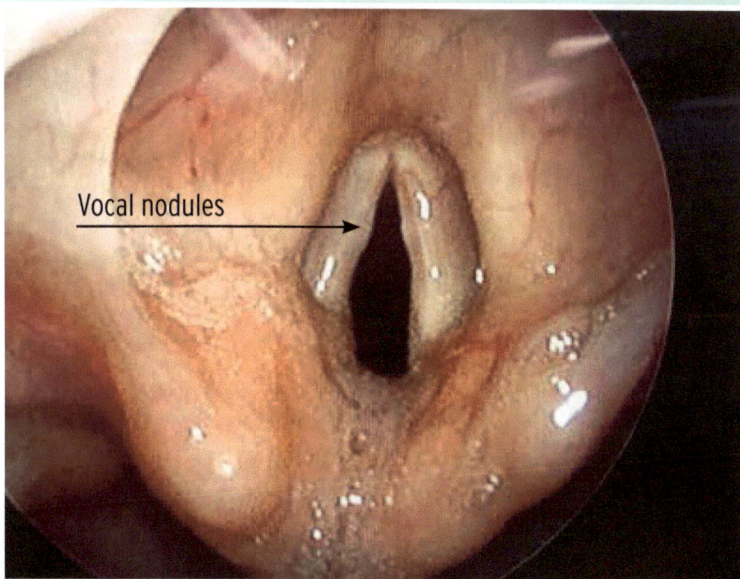

Vocal nodules

TRACHEOSTOMY

See Endnotes for comparison with Laryngectomy Page 114

- A **permanent** opening from the trachea to the lower neck.

TRACHEOTOMY

- A **temporary** opening from the trachea to the lower neck.
- Usually formed to bypass airway obstruction in the larynx or upper airway.
- Tracheostomy tubes come in various forms and sizes.

   1. Cuffed tracheostomy tube – this enables the lungs to be protected from secretions and blood passing down the trachea.

   2. Uncuffed tracheostomy tube maintains breathing passage open and allows some air to the vocal cords for voice production.

   3. Fenestrated tubes – allows air to pass through the larynx and allows voice production.

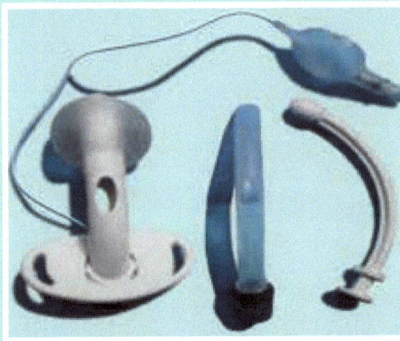

Cuffed and fenestrated tracheostomy tube with inner tube (for cleaning) and introducer

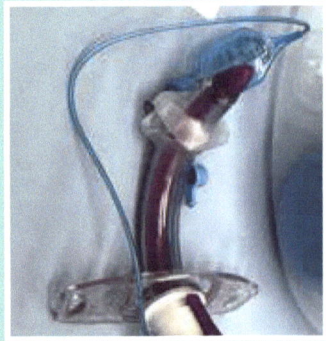

Cuffed tracheostomy tube with introducer

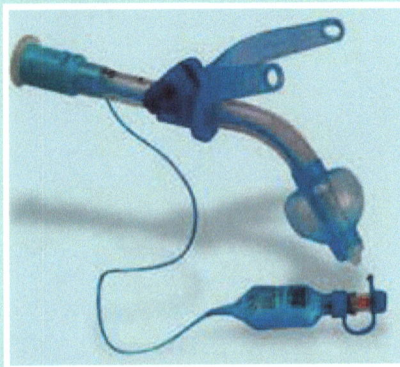

Adjustable tracheostomy tube for patients with thick necks

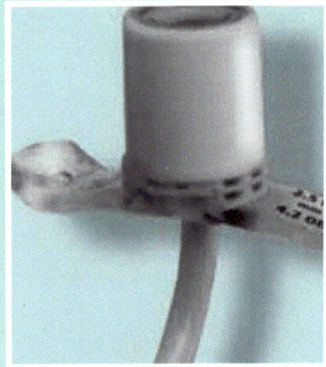

Paediactric tracheostomy tube showing internal and external size

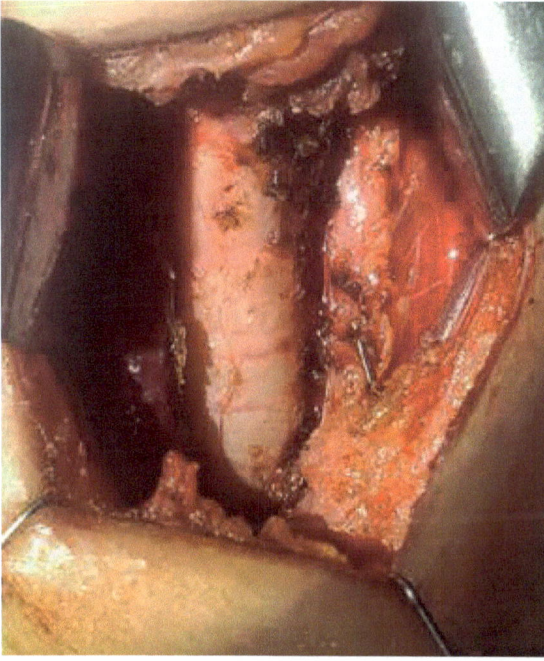

Trachea exposed showing the tracheal rings in the area for tracheal incision and tracheostomy

Photo taken during thyroid surgery

4

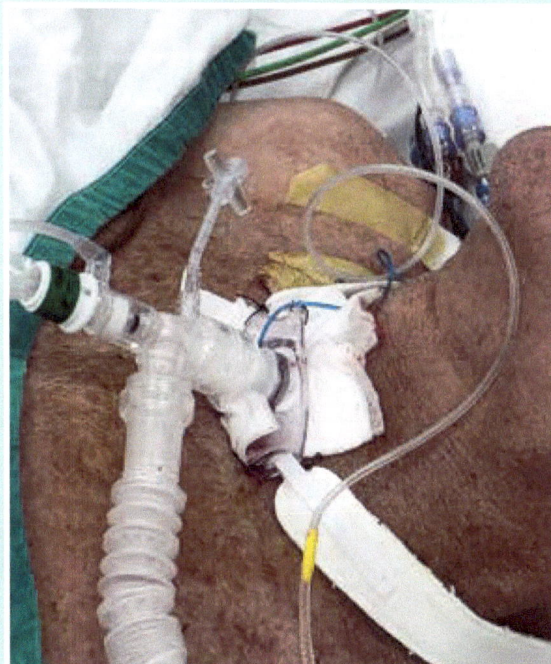

Patient in ICU with tracheostomy tube with ventilator connection and suction portal

CHAPTER 5

Paediatric Otolaryngology

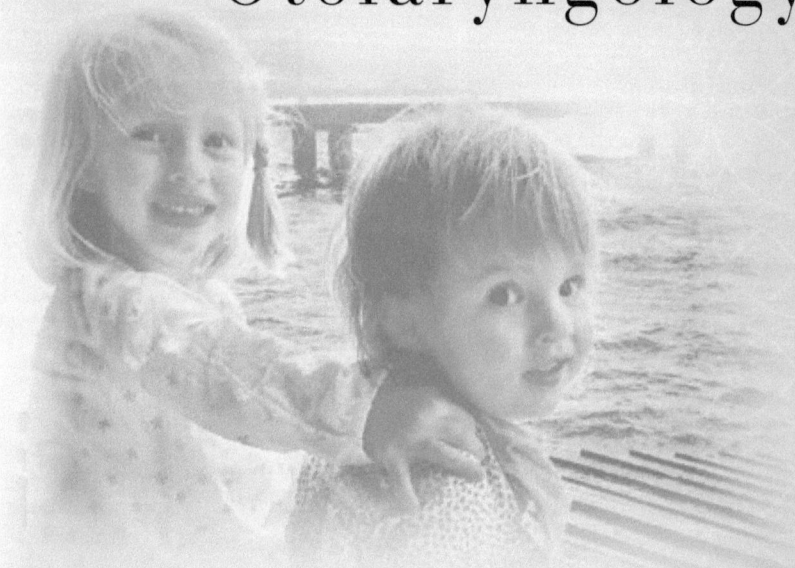

Particular emphasis here is placed on the throat and breathing disorders.

ACUTE OTITIS MEDIA (AOM)

Definition
- Inflammation of the middle ear space.

Epidemiology
- Common in infants and young children.
- 70 to 80% of infants have had at least one episode of AOM by the age of three.

Aetiology

- Most common causative agents:
  Streptococcus pneumoniae, Haemophilus influenzae;
  Moraxella catarrhalis.

Pathophysiology

- Due to Eustachian tube dysfunction.
  This leads to the air in the middle ear
  space being absorbed and negative
  pressure is a result. Secretions accumulate
  as they cannot drain, which eventually
  become colonized by bacteria,
  leading to inflammation and
  infection in the middle ear space.

Risk factors

- Young age.
- Day Care.
- Bottle feeding when supine.
- Tobacco smoke.
- Family history.
- Down Syndrome.

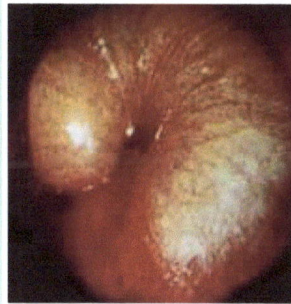

Acute otitis media
(about to rupture)

Clinical Presentation

- Otalgia, conductive hearing loss and fever.
- Otorrhoea when TM is perforated.
- If severe – vertigo, tinnitus and facial nerve paralysis may be present.
- In infants, symptoms include ear-tugging, irritability, vomiting,
  diarrhoea, fever and poor sleep.

Investigation

- Otoscopy: Bulging, erythematous TM. Perforation may be
  present with otorrhoea.

Treatment

- Analgesia: Paracetamol or NSAIDs.
- Antibiotics.
- If recurrent AOM, tympanostomy tubes can be inserted.

COMPLICATIONS

Extracranial	Intracranial
Mastoiditis	Meningitis
Cholesteatoma	Encephalitis
Ossicular chain necrosis	Intracranial abscess
Labyrinthitis	Sigmoid sinus thrombophlebitis

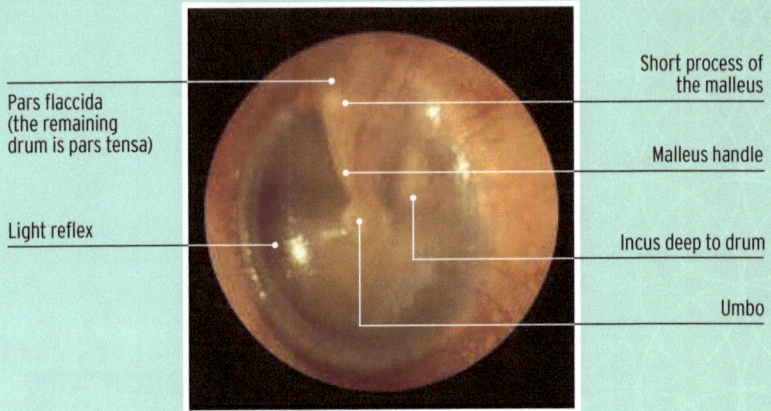

Pars flaccida (the remaining drum is pars tensa)

Light reflex

Short process of the malleus

Malleus handle

Incus deep to drum

Umbo

The normal eardrum

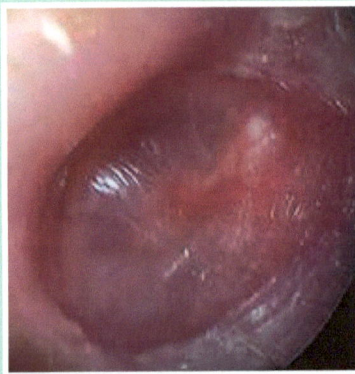

Middle ear effusion with air bubbles

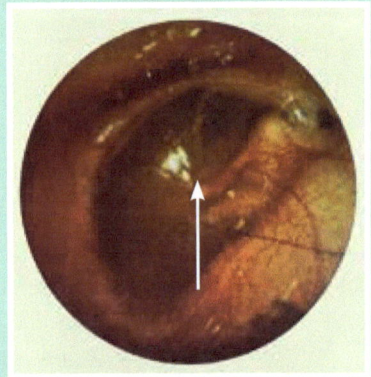

Arrow points to meniscus showing air / fluid interface

OTITIS MEDIA WITH EFFUSION (OME)

Definition
- Fluid in the middle ear without signs or symptoms of an acute ear infection.

Epidemiology
- Most common ear disease in young children.
- Generally precedes and follows AOM.
- More common in winter.

Risk factors
- Same risk factors as AOM.

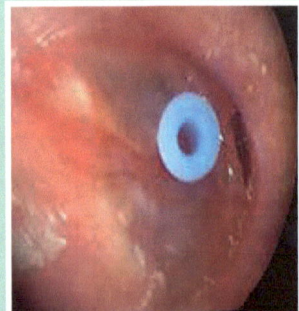

Ventilation tube in tympanic membrane

Clinical Presentation
- Conductive hearing loss.
- May have otalgia, sleep disturbance or tinnitus.
- Speech and language developmental delay can occur.

Investigation
- Otoscopy: Pale/vascular tympanic membrane with yellow fluid in the middle ear (occasional blue glue present), fluid level behind the TM may be seen, retraction of the TM.
- Pneumatic otoscopy: Decreased mobility of TM.
- Audiogram: Conductive hearing loss (often 30 dB of loss present).
- Tympanogram: Flat line (type B) – low volume.

Treatment
- Resolves spontaneously in the majority of cases.
- If persistent, surgery for placement of tympanostomy tube.

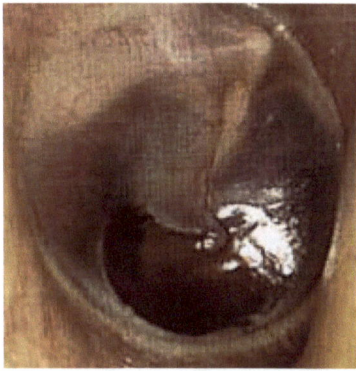

Middle ear fluid with retraction of the drum and yellowish fluid visible through the lower drum

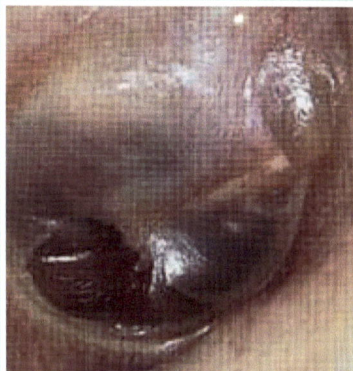

Same patient as adjacent photo following valsalva manoeuvre – note air bubble to the right with yellow fluid inferiorly (note also bulging of the pars flaccida)

5

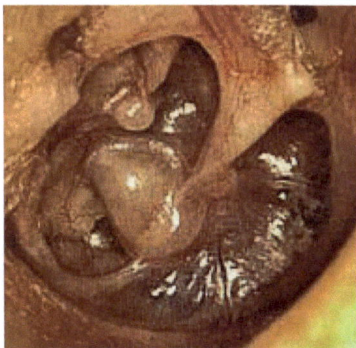

Retraction of the drum from chronic effusion

ADENOID HYPERTROPHY

Definition
- Hypertrophy of the **pharyngeal** tonsil (in the nasopharynx).

Epidemiology
- More common in children aged 3 to 6.

Clinical Presentation
- Nasal airway obstruction leading to mouth breathing.
- Nasal discharge, snoring, hyponasal voice and daytime sleepiness.

Investigation
- Endoscopy: Enlarged adenoid.
- Otoscopy: May show OME.
- Lateral X-ray: Adenoid shadow.

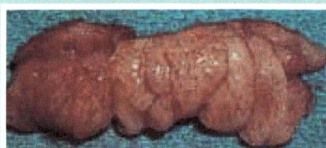

Adenoid - lymphoid tissue similar to a tonsil but without a capsule

Treatment
- Surgical: Adenoidectomy.

Complications
- Eustachian tube dysfunction leading to OME/AOM.
- Obstructive sleep apnoea.
- Orofacial developmental abnormalities due to chronic mouth breathing.
- Chronic rhinosinusitis.

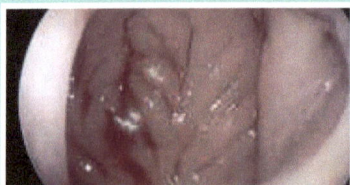

Normal small adenoid - seen at nasendoscopy

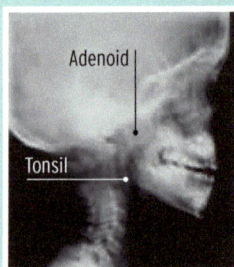

Lateral soft tissue X-ray of the pharynx

> **Key Point:** There are 3 different tonsils: 2 pairs (lingual and palatine) and a single adenoid.

ACUTE TONSILLITIS

Definition
- Acute inflammation of the **palatine** tonsils.

Epidemiology
- Incidence peaks in winter.
- Most prevalent in school children.

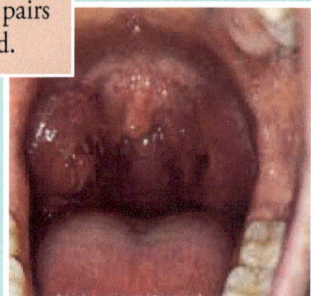

Streptococcal tonsillitis - compare a more exudative pattern on the next page

Aetiology
- Most common causative agent: Group A Beta-haemolytic streptococci.

Clinical Presentation
- Sore throat, fever, odynophagia, referred otalgia.
- Swollen, bright red tonsils. May have pus with other bacteria.
- Tender cervical lymphadenopathy.

Investigation
- Elevated WCC, ESR/CRP.
- Swab for culture and sensitivity.
- Rapid streptococcal test.

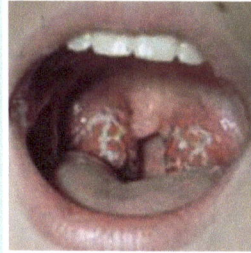

Acute tonsillitis

Treatment
- Analgesia.
- Salt water gargle for symptomatic relief.
- Antibiotics.
- Surgery: Tonsillectomy indicated for repeated infections.

Complications
- **Note: About 2% of patients may experience bleeding from the tonsil bed during the healing phase. If more than a spoonful of blood, admit for control of bleeding thus avoiding anti-coagulant medicine before and after surgery is important.**
- Acute rheumatic fever.
- Poststreptococcal glomerulonephritis.
- Peritonsillar abscess.
- Otitis media.
- Rhinosinusitis.

Key Point: Glandular fever with tonsillitis is characterised by very white spots over the tonsils. About ⅓ of cases will also have bacterial infection.

5

CHRONIC TONSILLITIS
- Charactarised by low grade tonsil discomfort and halitosis sometimes with mild upper neck lymphodenopathy.
- **Sulphur granules** with bad taste and halitosis are often noted.
- The symptoms are low grade and may recur over many years.
- Low grade fever is occasionally present.
- The typical cause is **actinomyces** (sulphur granules).
- These live in the tonsil crypts and excess colonies get pushed out into the oral cavity and pharynx.
- Definitive treatment is tonsillectomy. Antibiotics will only give temporary settling of the symptoms.
- If these calcify they become **tonsil stones**.

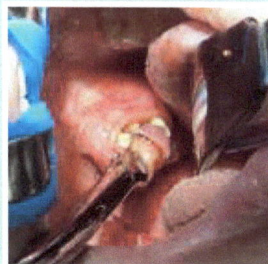

Chronic tonsillitis: Typical appearance of actinomyces which, if they calcify, become tonsil stones

PERITONSILLAR ABSCESS (QUINSY)

Definition
- Collection of pus in the peritonsillar space (outside the palatine tonsil capsule).

Epidemiology
- Most common deep neck space infection.

Aetiology
- Most common causative agents: S. pyogenes, S. aureus and anaerobes.

Pathophysiology
- Generally preceded by tonsillitis. Infection extends beyond the tonsillar capsule leading to peritonsillar cellulitis, followed by the formation of an abscess.

Risk factors
- Smoking.

Clinical Presentation
- Sore throat (unilateral), fever, 'hot potato' voice, drooling, trismus, referred otalgia (ipsilateral).
- Uvular deviation.
- May cause respiratory compromise if significant swelling.

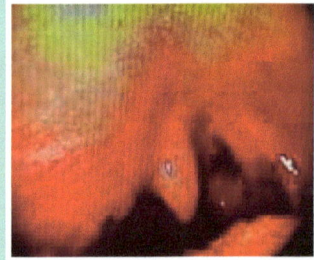

Quinsy – swelling is hiding the tonsil

Investigation
- Clinical diagnosis.
- May require CT scan.

Treatment
- Primary survey: ABC.
- Antibiotics and corticosteroids.
- Incision and drainage.
- Swab pus for culture and sensitivity.
- Surgical: Tonsillectomy if second presentation of quinsy or quinsy preceded by recurrent tonsillitis.

Complications
- Airway obstruction.
- Aspiration pneumonia.
- Sepsis.
- Mediastinitis.

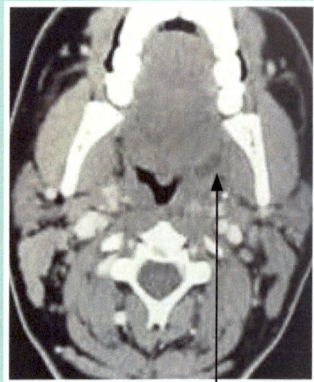

CT of left quinsy associated with enlarged left tonsil (Arrow pointing to loculated pus)

ACUTE LARYNGOTRACHEOBRONCHITIS (CROUP)

Definition
- Inflammation of the larynx and trachea that can extend into the bronchi.

Epidemiology
- Occurs predominately between ages 6 months to 3 years.

Aetiology
- Most common causative agents: Para-influenza virus (type 1 to 3), RSV, Adenovirus.

Pathophysiology
- The causative virus initially infects the nasal/pharyngeal mucosa and spreads to the larynx and trachea.

Risk factors
- Family history.

Clinical Presentation
- Usually begins with URTI symptoms (nasal discharge, nasal congestion).
- Dry, barking cough.
- Stridor, hoarseness, fever.
- If severe, can cause respiratory compromise.

Investigation
- Clinical diagnosis: Characteristic 'barking' cough.
- Frontal neck X-ray: Narrowing of the upper trachea (steeple sign).

Treatment
- Mild symptoms can be treated at home with airway humidification, antipyretics and oral hydration.
- Moderate to severe symptoms are treated with nebulised adrenaline, systemic corticosteroids and observation. Admission to hospital if no improvement or worsening after 3 to 4 hours.

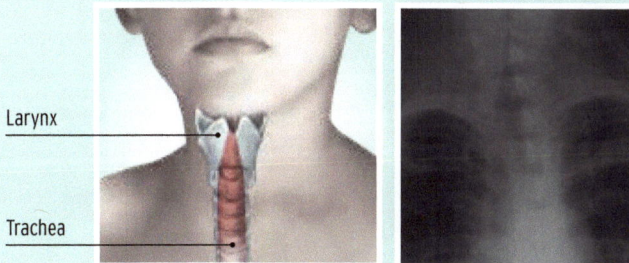

5

Larynx

Trachea

Drawing of neck showing trachea – see adjacent X-ray

Narrowing of upper trachea

ACUTE EPIGLOTTITIS

Definition
- Inflammation of the epiglottis and adjacent supraglottic structures.

Epidemiology
- Mostly affects children between 3 to 8 years of age.
- Incidence has declined since H. influenza vaccine was introduced.

Aetiology
- Most common causative agents: H. influenza, S. aureus.

Pathophysiology
- Infection generally spreads from posterior nasopharynx to the epiglottis and adjacent structures. Swelling of this region leads to turbulent airflow and may lead to complete airway obstruction.

Clinical Presentation
- Rapid onset and appears toxic.
- Fever, inspiratory stridor, hoarse voice, drooling, sore throat, dysphagia, respiratory distress.
- Tripod position: Sitting position with trunk leaning forward.

Investigation
- Clinical diagnosis.
- Lateral neck X-ray: Oedematous and enlarged epiglottis (thumb sign).
- Confirmed on direct inspection of the epiglottis only when securing the airway.

Treatment
- Examination and investigations may evoke laryngeal spasm leading to complete obstruction. Must secure the airway first.
- Intubation by anaesthesics.
- Antibiotics.
- Extubate once epiglottic swelling settles.

Key Point: Without immediate treatment, it can be fatal.

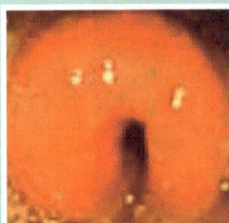

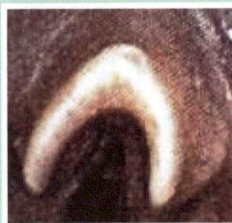

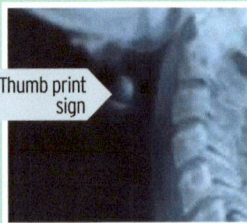

Thumb print sign

Acute epiglottis with normal comparison and the lateral X-ray showing thumb sign or thumb print sign

LARYNGOMALACIA

Definition
- Collapse of the supraglottic structures during inspiration.

Epidemiology
- Most common cause of congenital stridor.
- Generally resolves by 12 to 18 months.

Pathophysiology
- Supraglottic cartilaginous structures are abnormally soft causing them to collapse inwards during inspiration, resulting in airway obstruction.

Clinical Presentation
- Low pitched inspiratory stridor from birth or a few days from birth.
- Worse when supine.
- Can cause feeding difficulties.
- Rarely causes airway compromise.

Investigation
- Laryngoscopy: Collapse of supraglottic structures during inspiration will be seen. Also 'omega-shaped' epiglottis.

Treatment
- Majority of cases resolve spontaneously and only requires observation.
- In mild to moderate cases, medical management may include acid reflux suppression and high calorie formulas.
- In severe cases, surgery may be required: Supraglottoplasty.

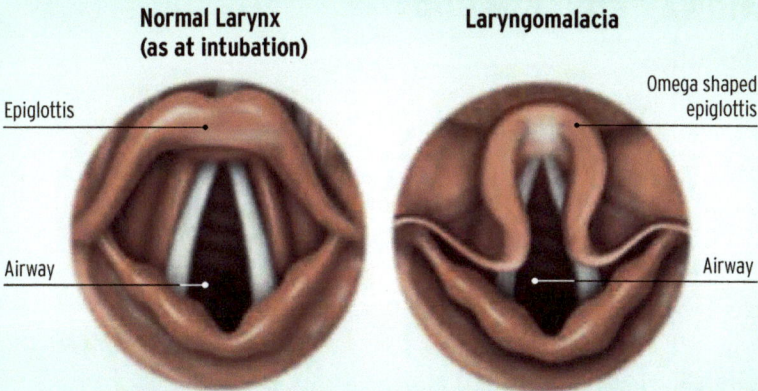

5

Normal Larynx (as at intubation)   **Laryngomalacia**

Epiglottis

Omega shaped epiglottis

Airway

Airway

PAEDIATRIC HEAD AND NECK MALIGNANCIES

These include:

Lymphomas.
Rhabdomyosarcomas.
Thyroid malignancy.
(NPC) Nasopharyngeal carcinoma.
Salivary gland malignancies.
Neuroblastomas and retinoblastomas.

} Often presenting as a lump in the neck.

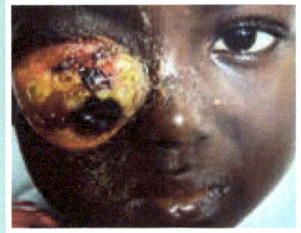
Retinoblastoma of the right eye

CLEFT PALATE AND CLEFT LIP

Clefts in the palate and lip arise during pregnancy.

There are varying degrees of these clefts which may affect one site only.

These give rise to feeding and speech difficulties and are often associated with middle ear effusion/infection due to alteration in muscle action on the Eustachian tubes.

Ventilation tube insertion is commonly required.

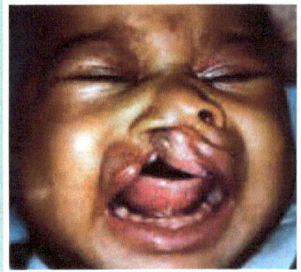
Cleft palate and lip

AIRWAY FOREIGN BODY

Definition
- Aspiration of a foreign body that can impair oxygenation and ventilation.

Epidemiology
- Majority of cases occur in children younger than 3 years.
- Common aspirated foreign bodies include peanuts, seeds, coins and paperclips.
- Majority of aspirated foreign bodies are located in the right main bronchus.

Clinical Presentation
- Symptoms depend on the size, shape and location of the foreign body as well as the age of the patient.

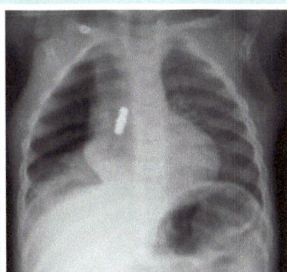

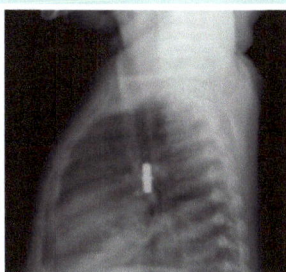

Foreign body in right main bronchus

- Most commonly present with cough, increased work of breathing and stridor, accompanied with unilateral wheeze and decreased air entry.
- Severe obstruction may present with respiratory distress, cyanosis and altered mental state that requires urgent intervention.

Investigation
- CXR.
- CT scan.

Treatment
- The foreign body should be removed as quickly as possible with rigid bronchoscopy.
- For unstable patients with complete airway obstruction, dislodgement using back blows/Heimlich Manoeuvre, should be attempted first.

Complications
- Atelectasis.
- Postobstructive pneumonia.
- Pulmonary abscess.
- Bronchiectasis.

Button battery at X-ray showing typical double edge

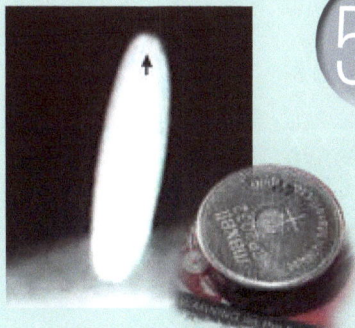

BUTTON BATTERIES
- If swallowed or in the nose or ear, this is an **EMERGENCY**.
  They can burn through the oesophagus in 2 hours and be fatal.
- If passed beyond the oesophagus they rarely give problems.
- The larger 20mm batteries are the most dangerous.
- Require urgent removal.
- See National Guidelines.
- Nil by mouth except for honey. Treatment includes 20mls every 10 minutes until taken to hospital/theatre.

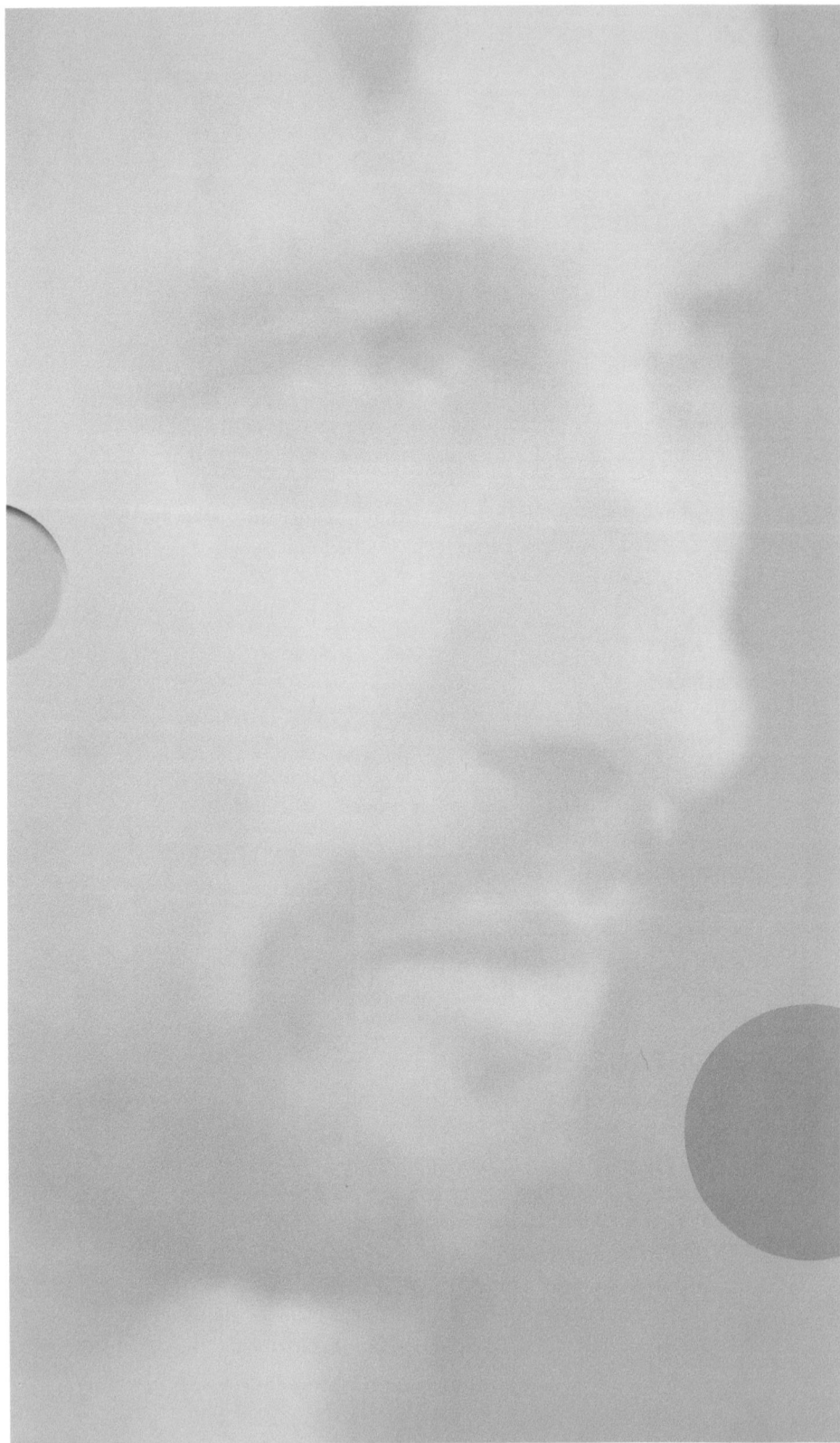

CHAPTER 6

General
Otolaryngology

Includes the structures of the face and the neck and the
conditions that commonly involve them, including:
Evaluation of neck masses.
Benign thyroid nodules (malignancy in latter section).
Deep neck space infections.
Salivary glands – stones, infections and benign tumours.

CONDITIONS REQUIRING URGENT ATTENTION

- Bleeding.
- Airway obstruction.
- Oesophageal obstruction.
- Button batteries.
- Sudden sensorineural hearing loss.
- Cellulitis.
- Visual changes with sinusitis (orbital or cavernous sinus involvement).
- CSF leaks.
- Penetrating injuries to the neck.
- Mastoiditis.

6

ANATOMY OF THE NECK

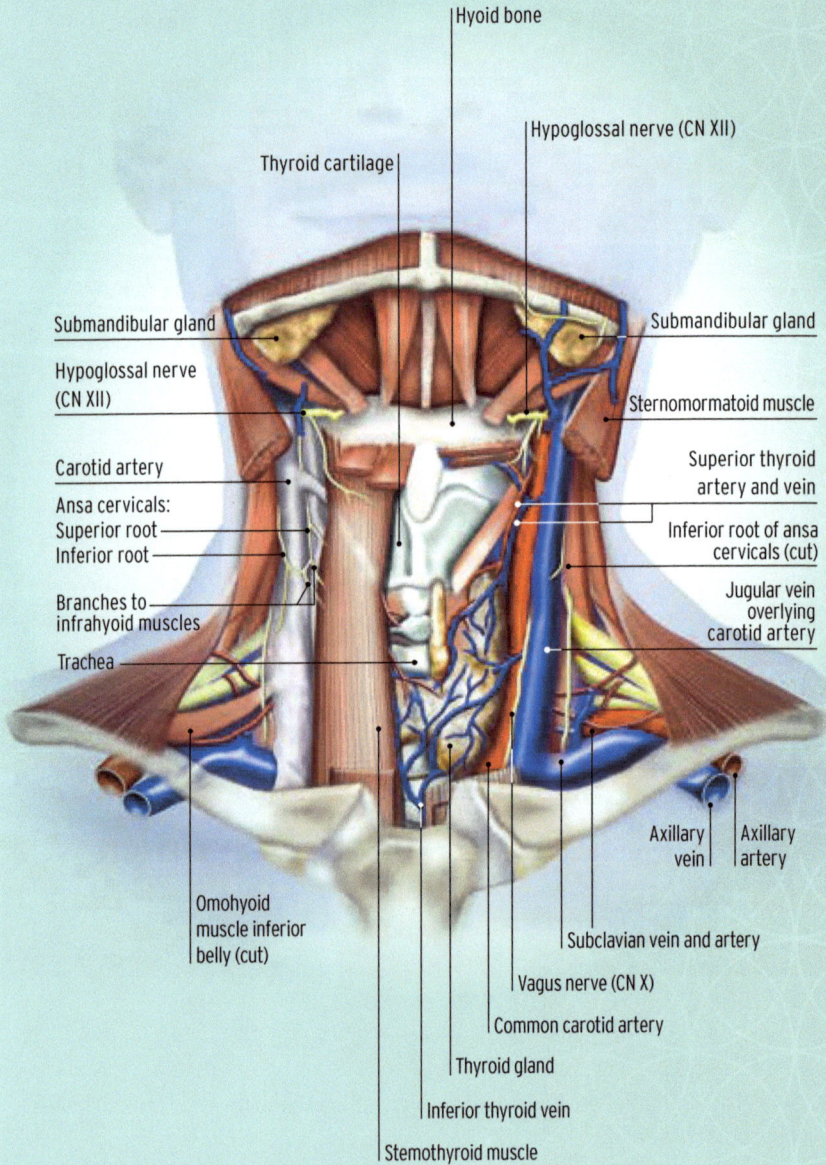

Hyoid bone

Hypoglossal nerve (CN XII)

Thyroid cartilage

Submandibular gland

Submandibular gland

Hypoglossal nerve (CN XII)

Sternomormatoid muscle

Carotid artery

Superior thyroid artery and vein

Ansa cervicals:
Superior root
Inferior root

Inferior root of ansa cervicals (cut)

Branches to infrahyoid muscles

Jugular vein overlying carotid artery

Trachea

Axillary vein

Axillary artery

Omohyoid muscle inferior belly (cut)

Subclavian vein and artery

Vagus nerve (CN X)

Common carotid artery

Thyroid gland

Inferior thyroid vein

Stemothyroid muscle

Fascial Layers of the Neck

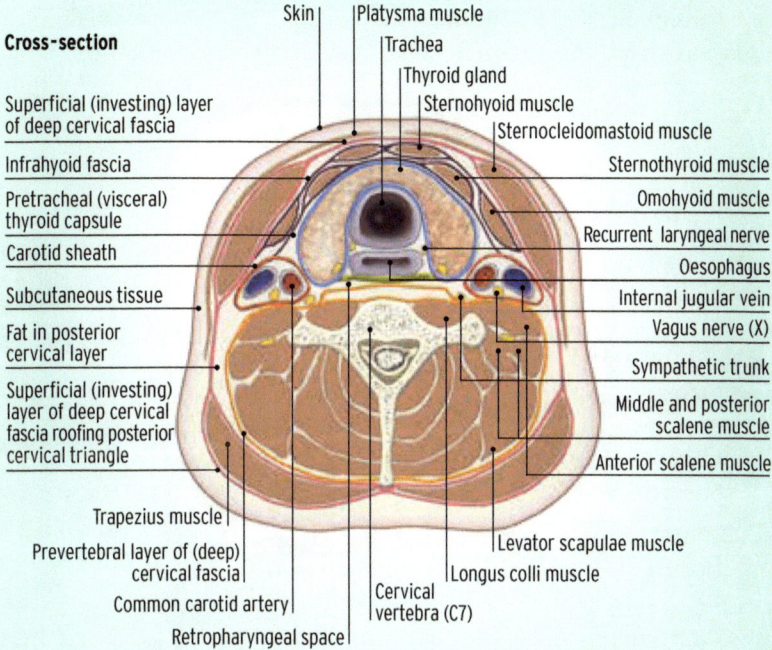

Cross-section

Skin | Platysma muscle
Trachea
Thyroid gland
Sternohyoid muscle
Sternocleidomastoid muscle

Superficial (investing) layer of deep cervical fascia

Infrahyoid fascia — Sternothyroid muscle

Pretracheal (visceral) thyroid capsule — Omohyoid muscle

Carotid sheath — Recurrent laryngeal nerve

Oesophagus

Subcutaneous tissue — Internal jugular vein

Fat in posterior cervical layer — Vagus nerve (X)

Sympathetic trunk

Superficial (investing) layer of deep cervical fascia roofing posterior cervical triangle — Middle and posterior scalene muscle

Anterior scalene muscle

Trapezius muscle

Prevertebral layer of (deep) cervical fascia — Levator scapulae muscle

Common carotid artery — Longus colli muscle

Cervical vertebra (C7)

Retropharyngeal space

Sagittal Section

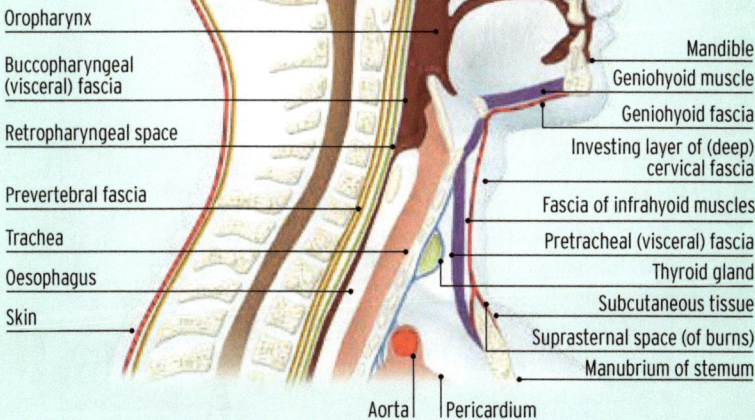

Oropharynx — Mandible

Buccopharyngeal (visceral) fascia — Geniohyoid muscle

Geniohyoid fascia

Retropharyngeal space — Investing layer of (deep) cervical fascia

Fascia of infrahyoid muscles

Prevertebral fascia — Pretracheal (visceral) fascia

Trachea — Thyroid gland

Oesophagus — Subcutaneous tissue

Skin — Suprasternal space (of burns)

Manubrium of sternum

Aorta | Pericardium

6

EVALUATION OF A NECK MASS

It is important to have a thorough history and examination when evaluating a neck mass. This will guide your investigations as the list of differentials are broad and can range from benign to serious causes.

Include a full history
- Size.
- Duration.
- Dysphagia.
- Hoarseness.
- Otalgia.
- Fever/sweats/weight loss.

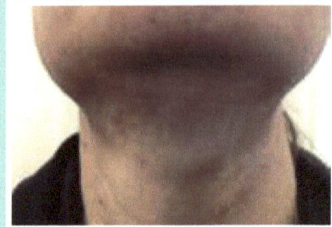

Thyroglossal cyst

Ask about risk factors
- Smoking.
- Alcohol.
- Other malignancy.
- Sun exposure.

Examination
- Inspect the neck.
- Palpate the neck.
- Is the lump:
  - Midline or lateral?
  - Hard or soft?
  - Fixed or mobile?
- Assess head and neck, skin and mucosa.
- Examine facial nerve function and for parotid swelling.

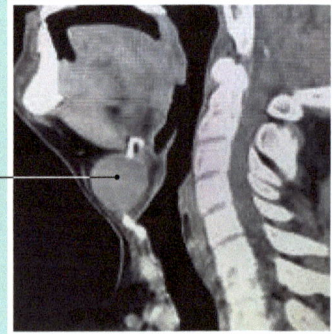

Thyroglossal cyst

Investigations
- CT scan + FNA of lump.
- For thyroid lumps – ultrasound and thyroid function tests.

DIFFERENTIALS
Congenital
- Thyroglossal duct cyst (midline).
- Branchial cleft cyst (lateral).
- Haemangioma.
- Laryngocele.
- Teratoma.

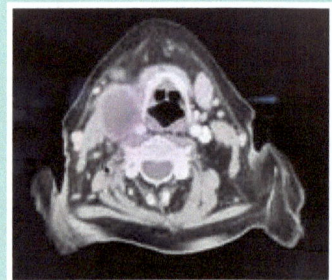

Branchial cyst

Inflammatory

- Cervical lymphadenopathy.
- Deep neck space infection.
- Abscess.

Neoplastic

- Metastatic disease.
- Thyroid tumour.
- Salivary gland tumour.
- Lymphoma.
- Vascular tumour.
- Lipoma.

BENIGN THYROID NODULES

- 95% of thyroid lumps are benign.
- Distinguishing the malignant 5% is important.
- Most thyroid nodules are adenomatous.
- Most are multiple.
- Usually 'cold' – non-functioning on scintigraphy.
- A few are 'toxic' – hyper functioning (hot on scintigraphy).
- When solid, the nodules capsule is well defined.
- The cystic adenomatous nodules contain haemorrhage with irregular internal walls and gelatinous fluid.
- Nodules may have micro or macro calcifications.

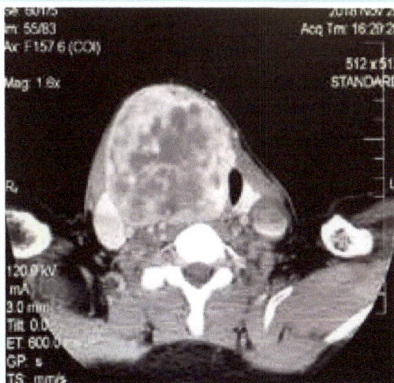

Benign thyroid nodules in the right lobe
Note: Small left thyroid lobe
Note: Goitre means thyroid enlargement

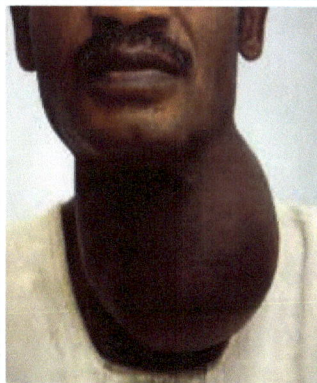

Benign thyroid nodules –
multi nodular goitre

- The most common adenoma is the follicular type – these are usually single and well encapsulated.
- They may be hypo or hyper-echoic and solid with the surrounding 'ring' called the halo sign.
- Parathyroid adenomas are occasionally ectopic within the thyroid.

Follicular adenomas are sub-classified by histological appearance of cellularity and colloid content into:

- Fetal (micro follicular).
- Colloid (macro follicular).
- Hurthle (oxyphil).
- Embryonal (atypical).

Presentation
- Asymptomatic.
- Noted by family member.
- Sometimes painful – if bleed occurs within the tissue.
- May compress the trachea.

Concern is raised by:
- Nodules >4cm.
- Firm.
- Fixed.
- Lymphadenopathy.
- Vocal cord palsy (hoarseness).

Treatment
- Treatment is determined by symptoms and size. Semi or total thyroidectomy being the main treatment options.

Key Point: The majority of nodules are benign. These need to be distinguished from malignancy. Thyroid nodules that are dominant or suspicious require ultrasound, FNA and thyroid function testing.

DEEP NECK SPACE INFECTIONS

Definition
- Two main types are retropharyngeal and parapharyngeal abscesses which can easily be overlooked if only oral examination is carried out. Ludwigs angina usually arises from skin or dental infections. These conditions may rapidly compromise the airway and need intubation or tracheotomy.
- Formation of an abscess between the planes of the deep cervical fascia.

Risk factors
- Dental infections.
- Trauma.
- URTI.
- IV drug use.
- Immunocompromised (e.g., diabetes, HIV).

Clinical Presentation
- Tender and erythematous neck.
- Associated with high fevers.
- Airway compromise, cranial nerve involvement and dysphagia may be present, depending on the location.

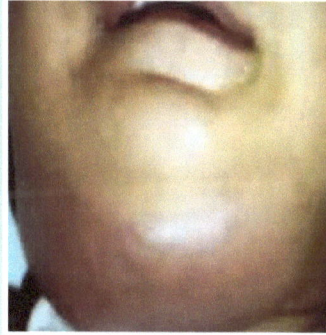

Ludwigs angina – swelling into the floor of the mouth may obstruct the airway at the tongue or pharyngeal levels

Investigation
- Neck X-ray: Lateral and AP.
- CT scan.

Treatment
- Prolonged course of antibiotics.
- Drainage of abscess.

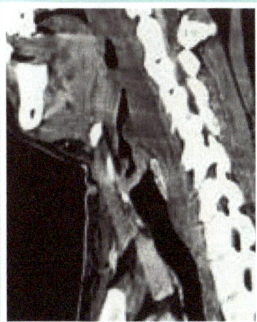

Developing retropharyngeal abscess also with epiglottic oedema (see thumb print sign)

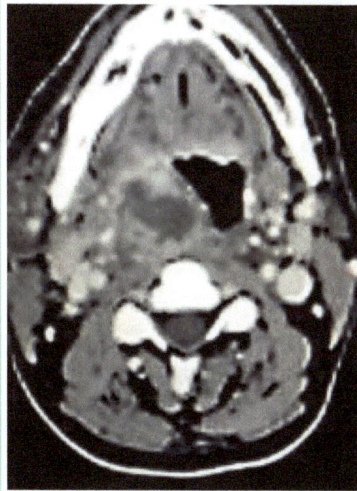

Retro pharynged abscess (axial view)

6

TRAUMA

Trauma to the head and neck region carries with it some specific issues especially as there are a number of nerves, vessels and related structures.

Blood loss is a key factor but maintenance of the airway is also essential.

There are a number of special considerations:

1. An apparent minor stabbing injury to the neck may give rise to bleeding from the major vessels.
To help with decisions of when to explore, the neck is divided into three regions: **A** Clavicle to cricoid. **B** Cricoid to mandible. **C** Mandible to skull base. Most injuries occur in region **B** which is the most readily accessible to explore.

2. A cervical spine injury may also be associated with a laryngeal fracture which if untreated may give rise to laryngeal stricture with obstruction. Look for surgical emphysema in the neck and loss of laryngeal prominence.

3. Hoarseness following injury to the neck may represent nerve damage (recurrent laryngeal nerve) or oedema or haematoma.

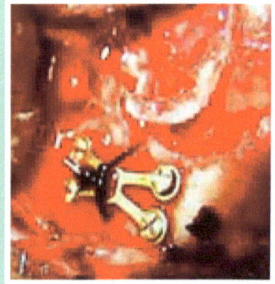

Laryngeal fracture plate

4. A laceration over the cheek may divide the parotid salivary duct resulting in a salivary fistula unless treated early by exploration and anastomosis.

5. A laceration to the face may transect the facial nerve branches – exploration and anastomosis may be required.

6. Depressed fractures of the frontal sinus may need elevation and plating.

7. Beware of orbital blow-out fractures and diplopia – muscle entrapment.

8. Check for CSF leaks in facial trauma.

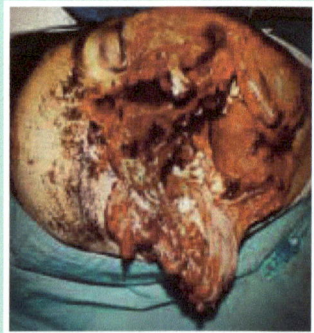

High powered gunshot wound

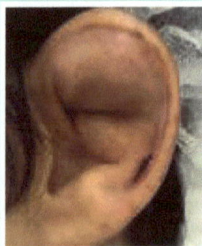

Auricular haematoma. Surgical drainage often required. Blood and serum collect under the perichondrium with trauma. Needle aspiration and open drainage may be required.

NASAL FRACTURES

Nasal fractures may involve the nasal bones and cartilages.

The need for fracture reduction is determined by cosmetic and breathing aspects.

Nasal bone fractures are best reduced when there is minimal swelling and before the bones re-unite, i.e., between 5 days after injury and 2 weeks.

At 3 weeks after injury, the healing is often too firmly healed to allow closed reduction and may need formal nasal bone refracturing. If only the cartilage is fractured, this is commonly left for 3 months to allow settling before arranging septal correction.

Check for adjacent fractures especially orbital floor fractures. Rhinoplasty may be required if the bones become set. This may involve bone cartilage and soft tissue modification.

DENTAL INFECTIONS

May give rise to cellulitis over the face and neck.

They may present as a lump in the neck and dental abscesses may discharge into the oral cavity through the gum or erode into the maxillary sinus and present as sinusitis.

The upper jaw/sinus infections have direct venous access to the brain – potential for brain abscess and meningitis.

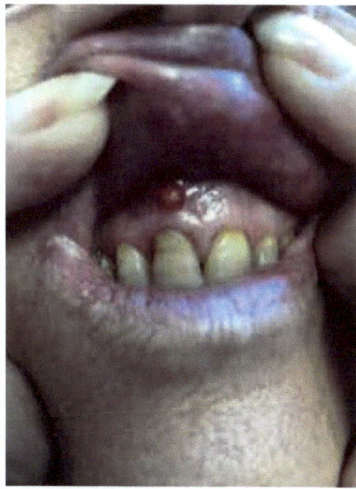

Dental abscess discharging through the gum

SALIVARY GLANDS

There are three pairs of major salivary glands (parotid, submandibular and sublingual) and hundreds of minor salivary glands that line the oral cavity and oropharynx.

The Major Salivary Glands

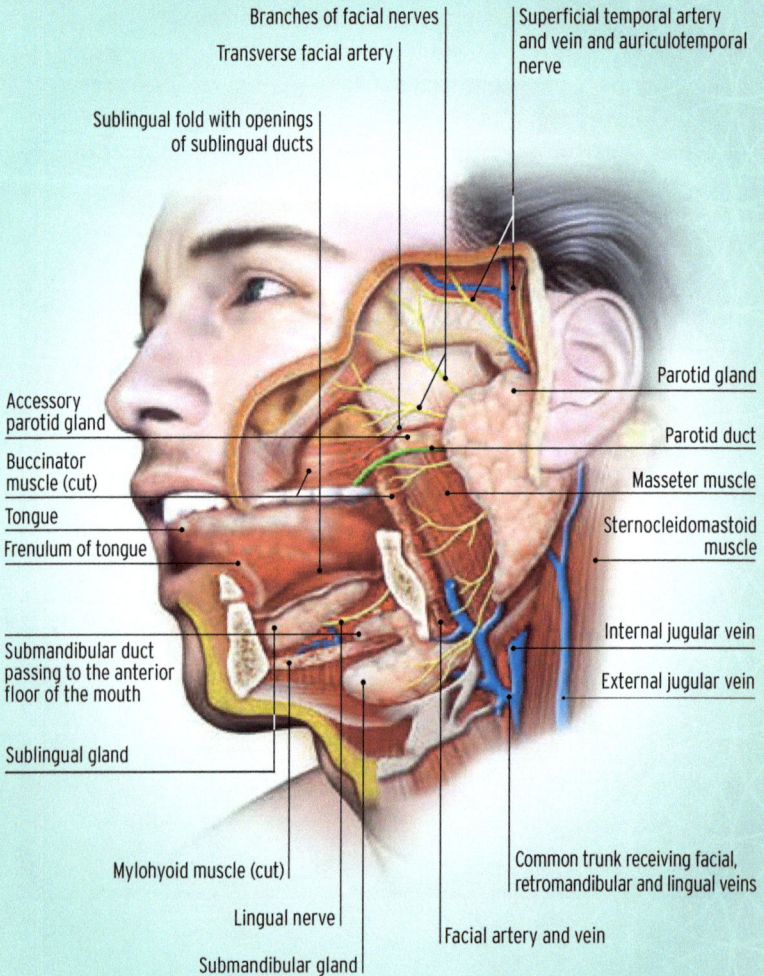

Branches of facial nerves

Transverse facial artery

Sublingual fold with openings of sublingual ducts

Superficial temporal artery and vein and auriculotemporal nerve

Accessory parotid gland

Buccinator muscle (cut)

Tongue

Frenulum of tongue

Parotid gland

Parotid duct

Masseter muscle

Sternocleidomastoid muscle

Submandibular duct passing to the anterior floor of the mouth

Sublingual gland

Internal jugular vein

External jugular vein

Mylohyoid muscle (cut)

Lingual nerve

Submandibular gland

Common trunk receiving facial, retromandibular and lingual veins

Facial artery and vein

SIALOLITHIASIS

Definition
- The presence of stones in any of the salivary glands or ducts.

Epidemiology
- The majority of stones relate to the submandibular glands.
- More common in men.
- More common in adulthood.

Aetiology
- Exact aetiology is unknown. Thought to be secondary to stagnation of calcium rich saliva. This can be due to local inflammation or injury to the gland/duct.

Clinical Presentation
- Pain and swelling in the involved gland. Sometimes can be painless.
- Eating or the anticipation of eating can incite a response.
- Stones may be palpable or seen at the duct orifices on examination of the oral cavity.

Investigation
- CT scan – gold standard.
- Ultrasound.

Treatment
- Majority of cases are managed conservatively (i.e., hydration, sialogogues, gland massage).
- NSAIDs for pain.
- Antibiotics if infection is suspected.
- Larger stones may require surgical intervention.

Complications
- Sialadenitis.
- Salivary gland abscess.

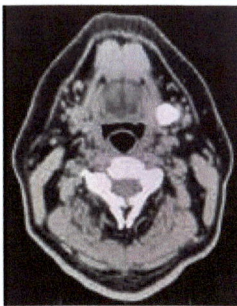

Left submandibular
duct /gland stone

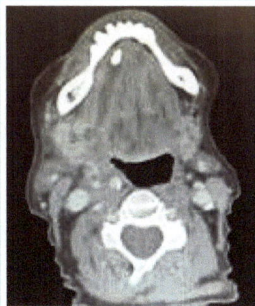

Right submandibular duct
stone with diluted duct

6

ACUTE SIALADENITIS

Definition
- Inflammation of any of the salivary glands.

Epidemiology
- Most commonly affects the parotid glands.

Aetiology
- Bacterial: S. aureus (most common), S. pneumoniae, S. viridans, H. influenza, S. pyogenes.
- Viral: Mumps, HIV, influenza, coxsackie.

Pathophysiology
- Due to obstruction or salivary stasis (usually in the ducts). This leads to bacteria ascending up to the affected salivary gland.

Risk factors
- Dehydration.
- Radiation and chemotherapy.
- Post-operative patients.
- Malnutrition.

Clinical Presentation
- Tender and swollen gland.
- Overlying erythema and warm to touch.
- Purulent drainage from the duct orifice of the affected gland.
- Trismus may be present.

Diagnosis
- Clinical diagnosis supported by imaging (US or CT scan).

Treatment
- Antibiotics.
- Analgesia.
- Hydration.
- Warm compresses and salivary gland massage.

Complications
- Salivary gland abscess.

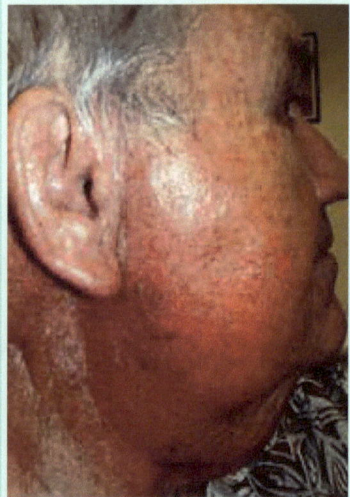

Parotitis – pain, swelling and often pus passing from the duct

BENIGN SALIVARY GLAND TUMOURS

These benign tumours generally present as painless nodules with no other symptoms. History and clinical examination, with ultrasound and fine needle aspiration biopsy (with CT scan or MRI) will give good information for diagnosis and treatment planning.

1. PLEOMORPHIC ADENOMA
Epidemiology
- These are the most common tumours of the salivary glands.
- The majority arise in the parotid gland.
- Occurs more frequently in women.

Clinical Presentation
- Painless, unilateral firm mass that slowly grows over years.

Investigation
- Ultrasound.
- FNA biopsy.
- CT scan/MRI.

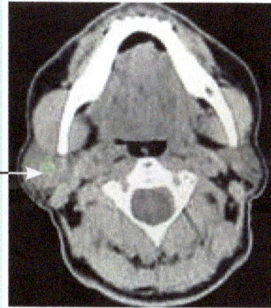

Benign tumour right parotid gland

Treatment
- Surgical resection with facial nerve preservation.

Complications
- Potential for malignant transformation.

2. WARTHIN'S TUMOUR (PAPILLARY CYSTADENOMA LYMPHOMATOSUM)
Epidemiology
- Second most common salivary gland tumour.
- The majority arise in the parotid gland.
- Almost all occur in males.

Clinical Presentation
- Painless 'soft' mass that slowly grows over years.

Investigation and Treatment
- Surgical treatment when symptomatic.

Complications
- Rare malignant transformation.

6

Key Point: No salivary gland mass should be left without a diagnosis. Do not carry out incisional biopsies due to risk of tumour implantation and facial nerve injury.

CHAPTER 7

Head and Neck Oncology

The majority of head and neck cancers are squamous cell cancers arising from the skin and mucus membranes with metastatic spread to the neck lymph nodes.

MALIGNANT TUMOURS OF THE NASAL CAVITY AND PARANASAL SINUSES

Head and neck cancers can arise in the nasal cavity, paranasal sinuses, oral cavity, pharynx, larynx, salivary glands and thyroid.

The initial evaluation of the head and neck cancer patient generally includes a thorough history and examination, endoscopy with biopsy, CXR and CT scan of neck. Additional investigations are based on clinical judgement and may include MRI and PET scans.

Nose and Sinus Tumours

Epidemiology

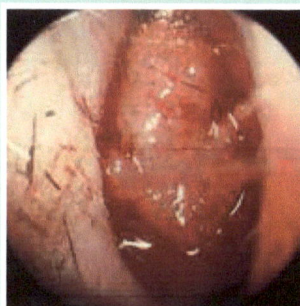

Malignant melanoma of the nasal cavity

- Rare tumours.
- Main site of involvement is the nasal cavity followed by the maxillary sinus.
- More common in males than females.
- Mean age: Sixth decade of life.

Aetiology

- SCC is the most common malignant tumour of the nasal cavity.
- Others include adenocarcinoma, neuroendocrine tumours and mucosal melanomas.

Risk factors

- Tobacco smoke.
- Occupational exposure: Wood dusts and glues.

Clinical Presentation

- Most patients present with advanced disease.
- Earlier symptoms include nasal obstruction and epistaxis.
- Late symptoms include facial swelling, orbital symptoms (diplopia, proptosis) and cranial nerve involvement.

Investigation

- Endoscopy.
- Biopsy.
- CT scan / MRI / PET.

Treatment

- Surgical resection and postoperative radiation.

7

Key Point: A malignant tumour should be a differential diagnosis in a patient with unilateral sinusitis unresponsive to treatment.

MALIGNANT TUMOURS OF THE ORAL CAVITY

Epidemiology
- More common in males than females.
- Mean age: Fifth decade of life.

Aetiology
- SCC is the most common malignant tumour of the oral cavity.

Risk factors
- Tobacco smoke.
- Alcohol.
- Tobacco chewing.
- HPV infection.
- Poor dentition.

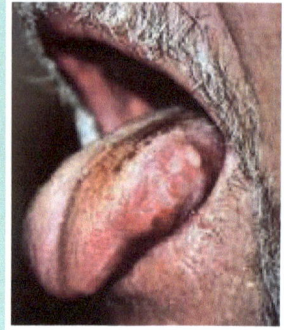

Squamous cell carcinoma of the left lateral tongue

Clinical Presentation
- Symptoms vary depending on location and size of the tumour. May be asymptomatic.
- Symptoms may include non-healing ulcers, odynophagia, halitosis and bloody saliva.

Investigation
- Biopsy.
- CT scan / MRI / PET.

Treatment
- Surgical resection of the tumour and postoperative radiation.
- Neck dissection may be indicated.

MALIGNANT TUMOURS OF THE NASOPHARYNX

Epidemiology
- More common in males than females.
- Mean age: Fifth decade of life.
- High prevalence in southern China.

Aetiology
- SCC is the most common malignant tumour of the nasopharynx.
- Lesser common tumours include: Adenocarcinoma, malignant melanoma, sarcoma and lymphoma.

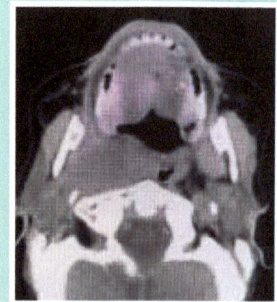

Nasopharyngeal carcinoma

Risk factors
- EBV infection.
- Tobacco smoking.
- Alcohol.
- Preserved foods.

Clinical Presentation
- Unilateral otitis media with hearing loss.
- Nasal obstruction with epistaxis.
- Cranial nerve involvement (diplopia, facial numbness).
- Neck mass (cervical nodes).
- May be asymptomatic in early disease.

Investigation
- Endoscopy.
- EBV antibody titre.
- CT scan / MRI / PET.

Treatment
- Radiation therapy (radiosensitive tumours).
- Neck dissection may be indicated.

Key Point: A malignant tumour should be investigated in adult patients with persistent middle ear effusion (with no past history of middle ear disease).

MALIGNANT TUMOURS OF THE OROPHARYNX

Epidemiology
- More common in males than females.
- Mean age: Fifth decade of life.
- Majority of tumours arise from the palatine tonsils or tongue base.

Aetiology
- SCC is the most common malignant tumour of the oropharynx.

Risk factors
- Tobacco smoke. • Alcohol.
- Tobacco chewing.
- HPV infection. HPV vaccination (Gardasil) is expected to lower the incidence of HPV related cancers.

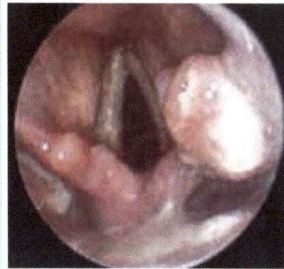

Oropharyngeal tumour

Clinical Presentation
- May be asymptomatic in early disease.
- Symptoms depend on location and size of tumour.
- May include odynophagia, halitosis, bloody saliva and trismus.

Investigation
- Biopsy. • CT scan / MRI / PET.

Treatment
- Surgical resection of tumour and postoperative radiation.
- Neck dissection may be indicated.
- For unresectable tumours, combination of radiation and chemotherapy.

MALIGNANT TUMOURS OF THE HYPOPHARYNX (LARYNGOPHARYNX)

Epidemiology
- Most tumours arise from the pyriform sinus. (Smuggler's fossa).

Aetiology
- SCC is the most common malignant tumour of the hypopharynx.

Risk factors
- Tobacco smoke.
- Alcohol.
- Tobacco chewing.
- Occupational exposure: Asbestos and coal.

Clinical Presentation
- Likely to be asymptomatic in early disease (large potential volume of the space).
- Symptoms include dysphagia, odynophagia and halitosis.
- Late symptoms include otalgia, hoarseness, dyspnoea and neck mass.

Investigation
- Endoscopy.
- Biopsy.
- CT scan / MRI / PET.

Treatment
- Radiation therapy for early stage cancer.
- Surgical resection for select cases.
- Neck dissection may be indicated.

MALIGNANT TUMOURS OF THE SALIVARY GLANDS

Epidemiology
- Malignant tumours may arise in any of the salivary glands (parotid, submandibular, sublingual and minor salivary glands).
- The majority of tumours arise in the parotid gland.

Aetiology
- SCC (also common site for metastatic SCC from skin of the head/face). In countries with high sun exposure and skin cancers, SCC metastasizing from the face and scalp can make this the most common malignant parotid cancer.
- Mucoepidermoid carcinoma.
- Acinic cell carcinoma.
- Adenocarcinoma.
- Adenoid cystic carcinoma.

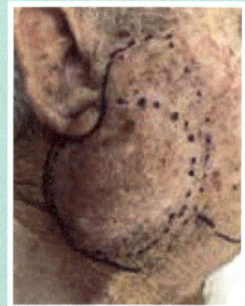

Right parotid gland squamous cell carcinoma

- Lymphoma.
- Carcinoma transformation in pleomorphic adenoma.

Risk factors
- Smoking. • Radiation exposure.
- Occupational exposure: Nickel, rubber, silica dust, asbestos.

Clinical Presentation
- Painful, fixed nodule.
- Rapid growth.
- Cranial nerve involvement (facial nerve palsy).
- Lymph node enlargement.

Investigation
- Fine needle aspiration.
- CT scan / MRI / PET.

Treatment
- Surgical resection of tumour and postoperative radiation.
- Neck dissection may be indicated.
- For parotid gland tumours, facial nerve preservation is not always possible.

MALIGNANT TUMOURS OF THE LARYNX

Epidemiology
- Second most common head and neck cancer (note HPV related SCC of oropharynx is most common).
- More common in males than females.
- Majority of tumours are located on the glottis, followed by the supraglottic region.

Aetiology
- SCC is the most common malignant tumour of the larynx.
- Others include undifferentiated carcinomas.

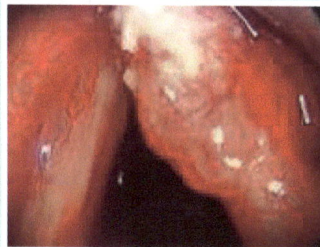

Carcinoma of the vocal cord

Risk factors
- Tobacco smoke.
- Alcohol.

Clinical Presentation
- Symptoms depend on the site of the tumour. May include globus sensation, dysphagia and constant throat clearing.
- For glottic tumours, hoarseness is most likely the initial symptom.
- For subglottic tumours, dyspnoea and stridor are likely.

Investigation
- Endoscopy.
- CT scan / MRI / PET.
- Microlaryngoscopy for biopsy.

Treatment
- For early disease: Laser excision or radiation therapy.
- Advanced disease may require total laryngectomy.
- Neck dissection may be indicated.

Key Point: Hoarseness lasting longer than three weeks should be investigated further with endoscopy.

LARYNGECTOMY

This is the removal of the larynx (voice box) usually to treat laryngeal cancer and sometimes trauma.

A stoma is created that joins the trachea to the anterior surface of the neck. No air passes from the lungs into the oral cavity. **Thus resuscitation is by providing support through the neck, not the mouth or nose.**

Speaking is made easier by the use of a speaking valve which is placed through the back of the trachea into the oesophagus. By placing a finger over the stoma and exhaling, air passes through the valve into the oesophagus and then into the oral cavity where it is modulated into speech.

An electrolarynx is a sound box which, when placed against the neck skin adjacent to the pharynx, can have the generated sound modulated into speech.

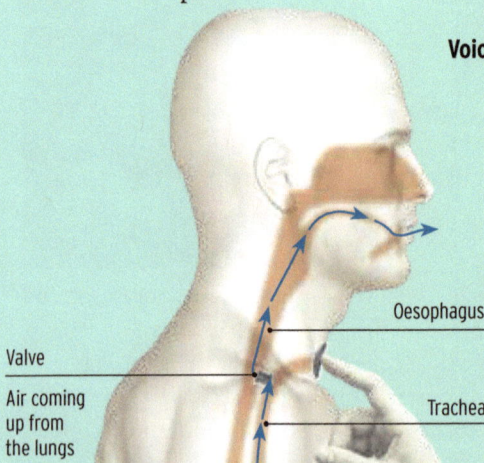

Voice Restoration

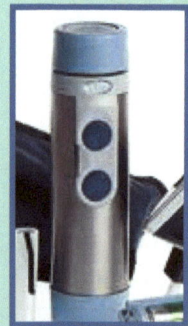

Oesophagus

Valve

Air coming up from the lungs

Trachea

Electrolarynx – sound generator

THYROID CANCER

Classification
- Papillary carcinoma:
    - Most common thyroid cancer (80%).
    - Good prognosis.
- Follicular carcinoma:
    - Second most common thyroid cancer (10%).
- Medullary carcinoma:
    - May be associated with MEN2 and have a familial association.
    - Lymph node involvement is common.
- Anaplastic carcinoma:
    - Most aggressive thyroid cancer-metastasis common at presentation.

Epidemiology
- More common in women.

Risk factors
- Radiation therapy.
- Thyroid enlargement.
- Family history.
- Autoimmune thyroiditis.
- Genetic disorder of MEN2.

Clinical Presentation
- Painless thyroid nodule or swelling.
- Larger tumours may present with dysphagia or hoarseness.

Investigation
- Ultrasound.
- FNA biopsy.

Treatment may include
- Surgery:
    - Total or partial thyroidectomy.
    - Neck dissection if positive lymph nodes.
- Radioactive iodine.
- Targeted chemotherapy agents (e.g., Vandetanib).
- Thyroid hormone replacement.

Thyroid Gland Relationships

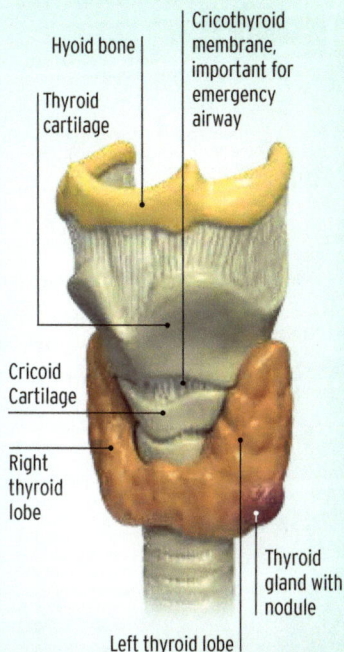

- Hyoid bone
- Thyroid cartilage
- Cricothyroid membrane, important for emergency airway
- Cricoid Cartilage
- Right thyroid lobe
- Thyroid gland with nodule
- Left thyroid lobe

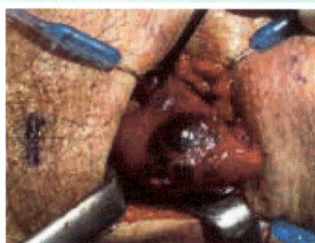

Papillory thyroid cancer - typically dark

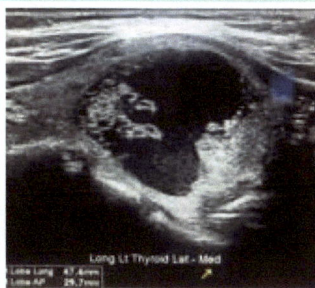

Complex thyroid module/cyst - may contain malignancy

7

SKIN CANCER OF THE HEAD AND NECK

Classification
- Basal cell carcinoma.
- Squamous cell carcinoma.
- Malignant melanoma (often referred to simply as melanoma).

Epidemiology
- Skin malignancies are common and a large proportion of these occur in the head and neck.
- Basal cell cancers are the most common and rarely spread but can be locally aggressive (Rodent Ulcers).
- Squamous cell cancers are more aggressive and may require local extensive surgery and neck dissection for lymph node spread.
- Melanoma is the least common skin cancer but is responsible for most deaths and spreads by lymphatic and blood making it less predictable.

Risk factors
- Sun exposure.
- Tanning beds.
- Prior head and neck irradiation.
- Immunosuppressive medications.
- Arsenic exposure.
- Fair skin.

Clinical Presentation
- Abnormal growth on the skin, which may be pearly, crusted, warty, ulcerated, mole-like and sore. It may bleed.
- In long standing moles, change is a warning sign of melanoma
  - ABCDE – asymmetry, irregular border, colour changes, diameter (>1cm), evolution.
- Melanoma may also present with an enlarged lymph node.

Diagnosis/Investigations
- Clinical exam and **excisional** biopsy.
- Fine needle aspiration cytology for any neck nodes.

Treatment
- Avoid excess sun exposure.
- Surgical excision with clear margins.
- May require neck dissection if positive neck nodes.
- Radiation therapy may be indicated in some circumstances (i.e., close/positive margins).
- SCC often metastasise from the head skin to the parotid glands and may spread along nerves.

- Melanomas are staged by their thickness (Breslow Depth thickness and Clark Level) into the skin layers. Thus shave biopsies are not appropriate. Sentinel node biopsies are often required for intermediate thickness tumours.

See explanation of T Staging for Melanoma on Page 113

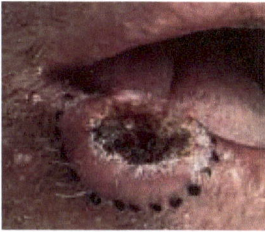

Squamous cell carcinoma of the lip (marking shows palpable edge not the surgical margin)

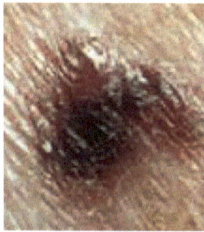

Malignant melanoma of the cheek

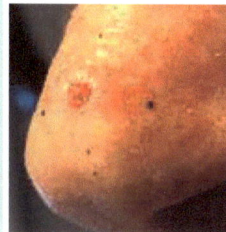

Basal cell carcinoma of the nose with pearly raised edges

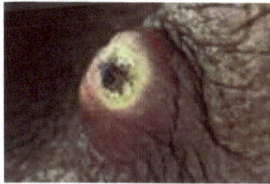

Beware the fungating cancer from the deeper neck – they can mimic infection

COMMON RECONSTRUCTION METHODS

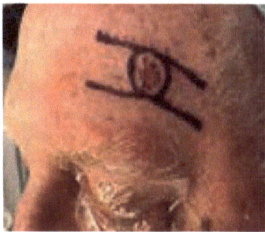

'H' flap

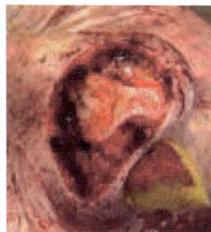

Excision site on nose for skin grafting

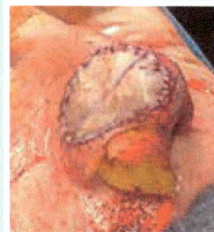

Skin graft to nose

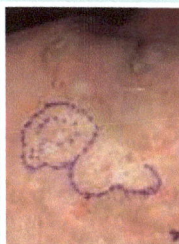

Tumour excision with bilobe flap repair

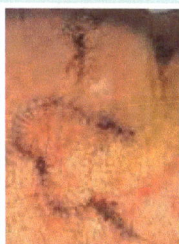

Metastatic SCC of the neck may arise from the following sites:

Nasopharynx (posterior to nose)

Oral cavity and tongue

Metastatic cancer from the scalp often presents in the parotid gland as a lump

Larynx

Virchow node

Oesophagus

Squamous cell cancers (SCC) in neck nodes arise from these common sites especially skin and mucosal surfaces

Stomach

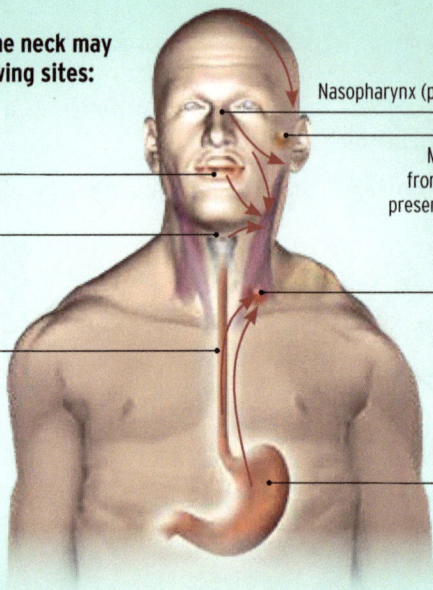

NECK DISSECTION

History

Radical Neck Dissection was the earliest surgical treatment for metastatic neck cancer – described by Crile in 1906. This involved removing all of the lymph node bearing tissues of the neck including the internal jugular vein, the sternocleidomastoid muscle and the accessory nerve. More recently, conservative procedures have been developed as it has become understood that:

1. Preserving non-lymphatic structures does not affect removal of lymphatic structures.

2. The location and size of the primary tumours of the head and neck have a predictable spread to specific nodal groups. This has allowed for a great number of surgical procedures for clinical variations.

General

Cancers in the Head and Neck commonly metastasize to cervical lymph nodes. Neck dissection refers to procedures that remove the fibro fatty contents that contain lymphatic structures which may contain metastases. Neck dissection is used in treatment of cancer of the:
- Aero digestive tract.
- Skin cancers.
- Thyroid.
- Salivary glands.

The Levels of the Neck

Note: The neck is divided into **6** lymph node levels to aid communication and treatment of disease.

If you understand level **3** then all of the others fall into place. Level **3** is triangular and lies from the posterior border of sternomastoid muscle to the omohyoid muscle and from hyoid bone to where the omohyoid muscle runs deep to the sternomastoid muscle.

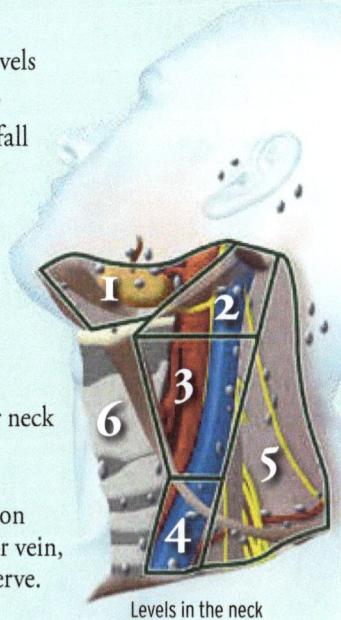

Terminology

- Radical Neck Dissection:
    - Is the key procedure to compare all other neck dissections.
- Modified Radical Neck Dissection:
    - Relates to preservation of one or more non lymphatic structures e.g., internal jugular vein, sternocleidomastoid muscle, accessory nerve.
- Selective Neck Dissection:
    - Relates to preservation of one or more groups of lymph nodes.
- Extended Radical Neck Dissection:
    - Relates to removal of one or more additional structures e.g., an additional lymph node group, carotid artery.

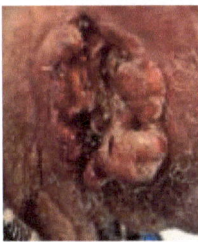

Levels in the neck

Untreated neck node cancer fungating through the skin

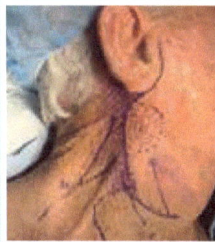

Planning for neck dissection

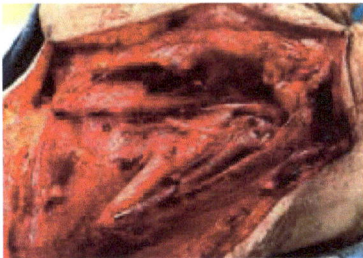

Dissected internal jugular vein posterior to the carotid artery with partially dissected sternomastoid muscle

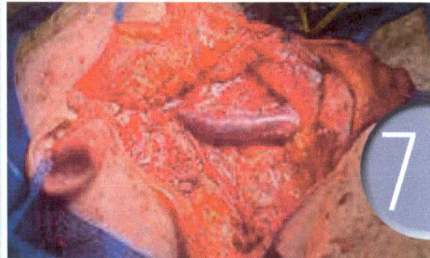

Neck dissection with removal of the sternomastoid muscle for cancer invasion of the muscle

DYSPHAGIA

1. Difficulty swallowing – liquid or food
Compare with **1.** Odynophagia – pain with swallowing (may occur with dysphagia) and **2.** Globus – the sensation of a mass in the throat.

2. Main subdivisions
- Oropharyngeal dysphagia – abnormality of initiation of the swallowing reflex in the oropharynx.
- Oesophageal dysphagia – abnormality of food bolus passing through the oesophagus.

> *Key Point:* The causes of dysphagia varies and treatment depends on the cause.

OROPHARYNGEAL DYSPHAGIA
Conditions that affect the throat muscles make it difficult for food to transit from the mouth to your throat and oesophagus which may lead to gagging, coughing or choking-related to aspiration into the trachea (may lead to pneumonia) or nasopharyngeal regurgitation.

Causes

1. Neurological disorder or damage especially stroke, brain and spinal cord injury.
- Parkinson's Disease.
- Multiple sclerosis.
- Muscular dystrophy.

2. Pharyngeal pouch (Zenker's diverticulum).
An out-pouching of the pharynx which gives dysphagia, gurgling, halitosis, coughing and throat clearing. Collects food and fluid.

3. Cancer – most commonly squamous cell carcinomas.

4. Scar formation from trauma, acid reflux, radiation.

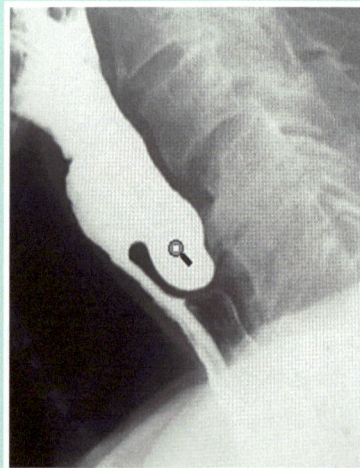

Lateral neck view during a barium swallow showing pouch with marker and division wall separating from the oesophagous anteriorly (Surgery to divide the division wall is called Dohlman's procedure)

OESOPHAGEAL DYSPHAGIA

Causes

- Oesophageal dysmotility.
- Oesophageal stricture.
- Achalasia – poor relaxation of lower oesophageal sphincter.
- Oesophageal tumours.
- Foreign bodies – beware button batteries and magnets
  EMERGENCY TREATMENT REQUIRED.
- Oesophageal ring.
- GORD – acid may give spasm and scars.
- Eosinophilic oesophagitis – the oesophagus becomes overpopulated by eosinophils and may be related to allergy.
- Scleroderma – gives scarring. Stiffening allows acid to back-flow into the oesophagus.
- Radiation for cancer may lead to scarring.

Causation factors

- Ageing.
- Reflux related to pouch formation.
- Iron deficiency anaemia – Plummer-Vinson Syndrome or Paterson-Kelly Syndrome associated with webs.

Complications

- Dehydration.
- Malnutrition.
- Aspiration pneumonia.
- Choking.

Oesophageal cancer

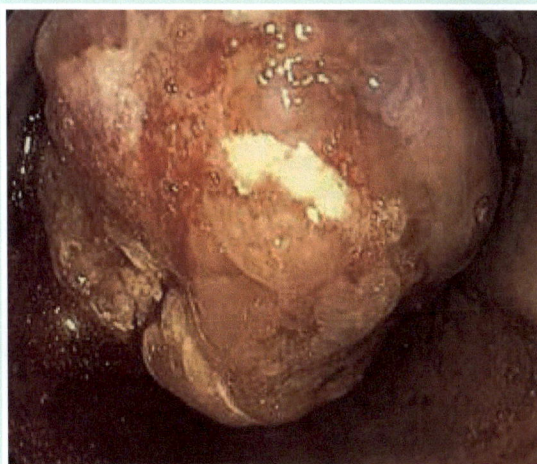

7

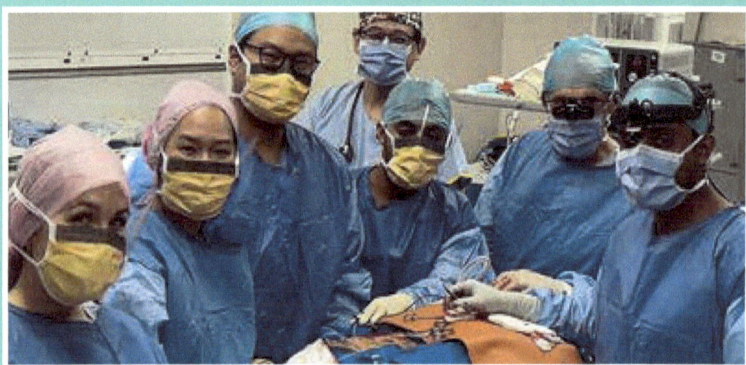

Training and learning involves the whole team

Endnotes

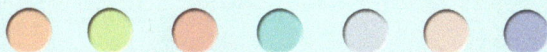

The speciality of OHNS is wide and constantly changing. It encompasses the conditions of the head and neck, some of which have medical and surgical treatments.

Sub-specialisation includes:

- Reconstruction of the head and neck.
- Oncological surgery.
- Otoneurology and skull base surgery.
- Facial plastic surgery.
- Thyroid/parathyroid and salivary gland pathology.
- Robotic surgery.
- Laser surgery.

Throughout the world, postgraduate training is arranged through divisions of the surgical colleges.

The key search word is Otolaryngology.

ABBREVIATIONS

ABC: Airway, Breathing and Circulation
ABCDE: Airway, Breathing, Circulation, Disability, Exposure
AC: Air Conduction
ANA: Antinuclear Antibodies
AOM: Acute Otitis Media
AP: Anterior/Posterior
ABR: Auditory Brain Stem Response
BAHA: Bone Anchored Hearing Aid
BC: Bone Conduction
BCC: Basal Cell Carcinoma
BPPV: Benign Paroxysmal Positional Vertigo

Abbreviations continued:

CHL: Conductive Hearing Loss
CMV: Cytomegalovirus
CN: Cranial Nerve
CNS: Central Nervous System
CRP: C-Reactive Protein
CSF: Cerebrospinal Fluid
CT: Computerised Tomography
CVA: Cerebrovascular Accident
  (stroke)
CXR: Chest X-ray
DCR: Dacryocystorhinostomy
EAC: External Auditory Canal
EBV: Epstein-Barr Virus
ED: Emergency Department
ESR: Erythrocyte Sedimentation Rate
FBC: Full Blood Count
FESS: Functional Endoscopic Sinus Surgery
FNA: Fine Needle Aspiration
GORD: Gastro-oesophageal Reflux Disease
HIV: Human Immunodeficiency Virus
HPV: Human Papilloma Virus
HSP: Heat Shock Protein
ICU: Intensive Care Unit
IgE: Immunoglobulin
IV: Intravenous
MEN2: Multiple Endocrine Neoplasia Type 2
MHL: Mixed Hearing Loss
MRI: Magnetic Resonance Imaging
NICU: Neonatal Intensive Care Unit
NPC: Nasopharyngeal Carcinoma
NPE: Nasopharyngeal Endoscopy
NSAIDs: Non-steroidal Anti-inflammatory Drugs
OE: Otitis Externa
OHNS: Otolaryngology, Head and Neck Surgery
OME: Otitis Media with Effusion
PCL: Papillary Cystadenoma Lymphomatosum
PET: Positron Emission Tomography
RSV: Respiratory Syncytial Virus
SCC: Squamous Cell Carcinoma
SNHL: Sensorineural Hearing Loss

T Staging: Tumour Staging
Tis: Tumour in situ
TM: Tympanic Membrane
TMJ: Temporomandibular Joint
TNM: Tumour Node Metastases
URTI: Upper Respiratory Tract
  Infection
US: Ultrasound
VOR: Vestibular Ocular Reflex
WCC: White Cell Count

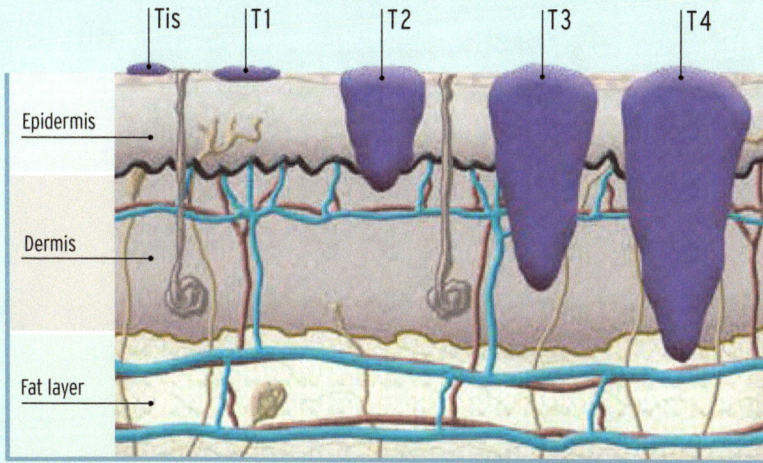

Tis   T1   T2   T3   T4

Epidermis

Dermis

Fat layer

THE T STAGING FOR MELANOMA *Following on from Page 105*

Melanomas and other cancers are classified by the TNM Staging System (T for Tumour size, N for Nodes in adjacent area and M for distant Metastases).

In melanoma prior to the TNM System, the Breslow (thickness of the tumour) and Clark Systems (level of skin involvement) were the key ways of staging melanoma growth.

The TNM System has 6 main stages for melanoma thickness, (Tis to T4).

Tis – melanoma *in situ.*

T0 – No melanoma cells at the primary site.

T1 ≤ 1 mm.
Divided in (a) – where < 0.8 mm and not ulcerated.
           (b) – either < 0.8 mm with ulceration.
              – or < 0.8 mm–1 mm with or without ulceration.

T2 melanoma 1–2 mm thick.

T3 2–4 mm thick.

T4 > 4 mm thick.

T2 and T4 are also subdivided into (a) without ulceration and (b) with ulceration.

COMPARISON - TRACHEOSTOMY AND LARYNGECTOMY

Following on from Page 68

Tracheostomy

Larynx still present (maybe narrow).

Upper airway intact.

In emergency – can give oxygen via nose or mouth and intubation could be attempted.

Fitted with tracheostomy tube Speaking possible by occluding tracheostomy tube if space allows air to pass up to vocal cords.

Mainly for airway obstruction or prolonged ventilation and suction.

Can be short or long term.

Laryngectomy

Larynx with vocal cords have been removed at surgery.

The trachea is now attached and open to the neck.

There is no connection between the mouth and nose to the trachea and lungs.

May or may not wear a tube to maintain the stoma open.

Electrolarynx or voice prosthesis allows speech.

Permanent airway.

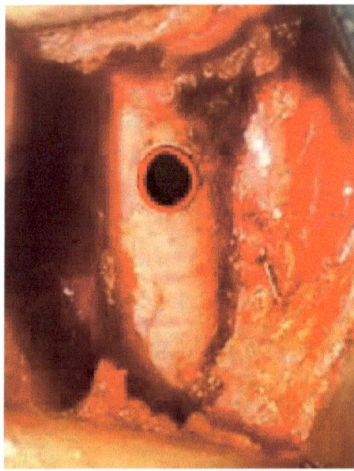

In tracheostomy a hole is opened into the trachea. This hole is in line with an opening in the skin.

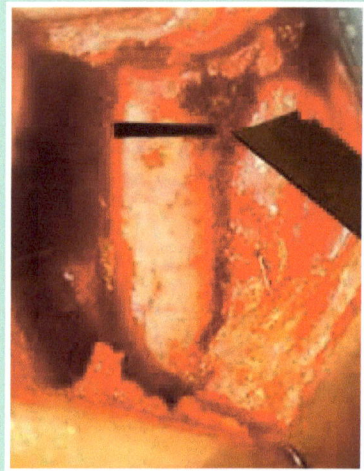

In laryngectomy the trachea is divided across the black line to allow the larynx above to be removed. Then the trachea is turned forward and sutured to the skin of the neck.

Cross-section of the Cochlea

Following on from Page 23

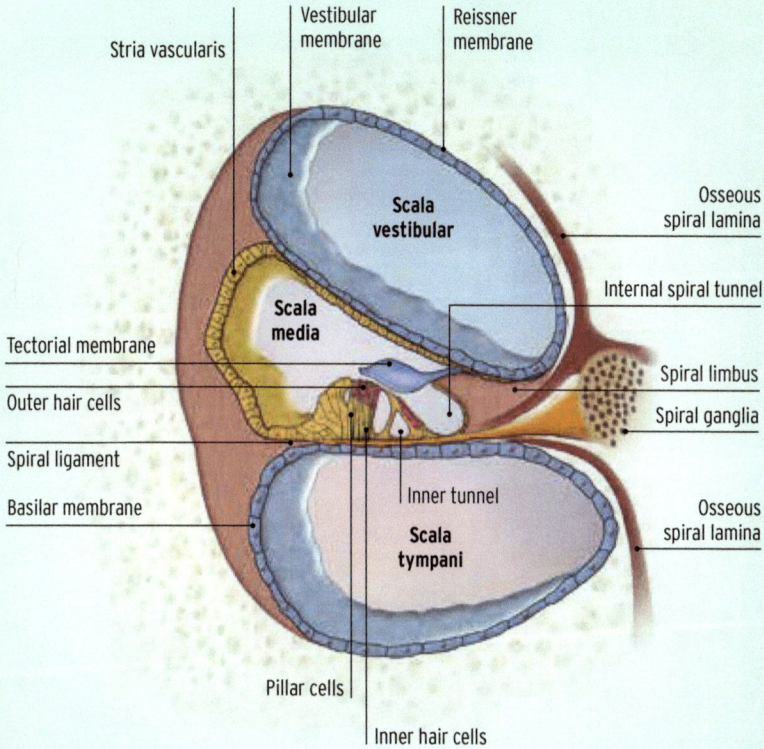

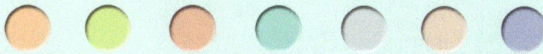

Labels:
- Stria vascularis
- Vestibular membrane
- Reissner membrane
- Scala vestibular
- Osseous spiral lamina
- Internal spiral tunnel
- Scala media
- Tectorial membrane
- Spiral limbus
- Outer hair cells
- Spiral ganglia
- Spiral ligament
- Inner tunnel
- Basilar membrane
- Scala tympani
- Osseous spiral lamina
- Pillar cells
- Inner hair cells

Notes

www.ingramcontent.com/pod-product-compliance
Lightning Source LLC
Chambersburg PA
CBHW041005210326
41597CB00001B/15